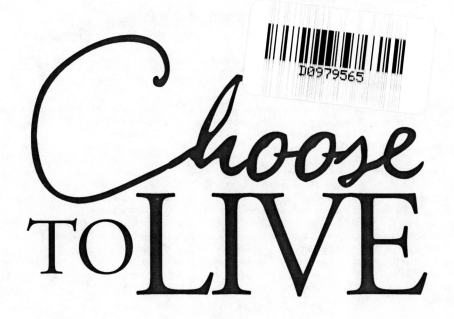

Choose TO LIVE

Our Journey From Late Stage Cancers to Vibrant Health

JOYCE O'BRIEN

EXPERT ACADEMY PRESS
an imprint of Morgan James Publishing
New York

Choose TO LIVE
OUR JOURNEY FROM LATE STAGE CANCERS TO VIBRANT HEALTH
by JOYCE O'BRIEN

ISBN 978-1-60037-836-2 (paperback)

Library of Congress Control Number: 2010936528

Published by:

EXPERT ACADEMY PRESS
an imprint of Morgan James Publishing
The Entrepreneurial Publisher
5 Penn Plaza, 23rd Floor
New York City, New York 10001
(212) 655-5470 Office
(516) 908-4496 Fax
www.MorganJamesPublishing.com

Cover photo by:
Jules Helm
juleshelm@juleshelm.com

Cover Design by:
Rachel Lopez
rachel@r2cdesign.com

Interior Design by:
Bonnie Bushman
bbushman@bresnan.net

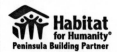

In an effort to support local communities, raise awareness and funds, Morgan James Publishing donates one percent of all book sales for the life of each book to Habitat for Humanity.
Get involved today, visit
www.HelpHabitatForHumanity.org.

DEDICATION

For my mom, our angel,
who carried us through on her wings.

RAVE REVIEWS

Like many charming young couples, Joyce and Kevin O'Brien apparently "had it all"—successful careers and a loving marriage—until that dream took on the quality of a nightmare when they were both, almost simultaneously, diagnosed with life-threatening conditions. Abruptly, their lives were filled with such despair that most people would have given up.

For Joyce and Kevin, however, this was not the end of their journey but the beginning. By recognizing their own power and the miracles that bless each and every one of us (if only we open our eyes to see them), Joyce and Kevin began the process of recovery. Often heartbreaking and frequently exhilarating, this remarkable story reminds each of us just what is possible in our own life— through determination, love, faith, and perseverance.

Having produced many stories over the years for Diane Sawyer, Charlie Rose, and Charles Kuralt, I've been associated with countless inspiring tales of individuals who overcame adversity in many forms, but I've never encountered a story quite like this. Without exaggeration, this is one of the most moving and inspiring books I've ever read.

—Tom Martin
President, Tom Martin Media, LLC

"Miracles happen when you know their secrets, Joyce and Kevin have a message everyone needs to hear. Read on to discover their secrets."

—Steven Sadleir
Director of the Self Awareness Institute, Best-selling author

O'Brien's journey from living the dream life of a thirty-something successful professional to the nightmare of her and her husband having advanced cancer is a roller coaster ride packed with emotions. Her passion for life jumps off the pages, and even in her darkest hour, her sense of humor shines through!

—JJ Virgin PhD, CNS
Celebrity Wellness Expert, Author of *Six Weeks to Sleeveless and Sexy*,
President of the National Association of Nutrition Professionals

It's not a book, but a black hole that sucks you in, wreaks havoc with your emotions, and then lets you out on the other side satisfied, inspired, and in awe of the human potential.

—Alex Lubarsky, CEO
Health Media Group, Inc.

O'Brien's path to becoming cancer free was not an easy one—she was diligent and unrelenting in her commitment to get well. She did everything she was told and more: she bravely ventured into an unconventional new world and never let go of hope, and as a reward for her determination, she and her husband beat all the odds.

—Richard Linchitz, MD
Board of Directors, International Organization of IPT Physicians (IOIP),
Board of Directors, International College of Integrative Medicine, (ICIM)
Board of Directors, American College for Advancement in Medicine (ACAM)

Truly one of the most inspirational books I have read. Joyce and Kevin O'Brien's remarkable story is told with humor and heart and stands as a testament to the triumph of human spirit. Nearly everyone has been touched by cancer in some way. Choose to Live! *provides a very real insight to the disease and, more importantly, serves as a valuable resource for anyone facing a life challenge—or can be passed on to someone who is. A must-read.*

—Dottie Galliano, President, Renaissance Media

FOREWORD

After reading Joyce's book and thinking about the title, I was reminded of a Biblical message: when life and death are placed before us, we are to choose life. By that, I do not mean merely to try to avoid dying, but to choose to live a meaningful life involving us in a demonstration of our love for ourselves and others. When we live that way, our body knows we love our life. It then does all it can to sustain us, heal our afflictions and wounds, and keep us healthy.

When we do not love our life and body, our body interprets the messages it gets as our desire to end our lives. It tries hard to please us, as Monday morning demonstrates with its increased incidence of major diseases and suicides. *Choose to Live* demonstrates what its title says. It lives the message. It can show you how to turn a curse into a blessing and can, through life's difficulties—or what I call the labor pains of life—help you be reborn to the life you desire. It restores your ability to enjoy the emotional and physical benefits that come with the new life. Then your problem becomes a gift and wake-up call, because it provides you with a new beginning.

Life is not unfair, but it is difficult. We all need help and coaching so that we are prepared for the difficulties we will all encounter. If we have not been taught at an early age by the authority figures in our lives, we have to learn from others and reparent ourselves. It is then that we establish self-worth and the desire to heal our lives. We can learn to face the sun and not see the shadows, as Joyce shows us, and not let a doctor's *words* become *swords* which can kill instead of cure us. There is no secret to survival. We can learn from others who exceed all expectations of what survival behavior is and how to accomplish it. That is what this book is about. Yes, it is a story, but stories are often the truest truth of all, and we can learn from them.

And yet, doctors rarely ask patients *why* they are doing better than expected, so that they might pass the word along. They think you are lucky or have a spontaneous remission when it is really self-induced healing. Just as hunger leads us to seek nourishment, our physical and emotional problems can lead us to nourish our lives. Then we derive the benefits that come when we create our authentic lives and no longer live those imposed on us by others.

One must love oneself to accomplish this. Information does not solve the world's problems, or the individual's, if it is not accomplished by inspiration. To derive the benefits inherent in reading this book, you have to care about yourself and not be fearful of guilt, shame, and blame if you don't have the result you desire. The question is, are you willing to give it a try, participate in your life and health, and take responsibility for your choices and actions? It isn't about not dying—death is inevitable. It is about participating in, and taking responsibility for, your life.

If you value yourself and do not fear failure, you are what I call a "respant," or "responsible participant," so read on. If, on the other hand, you are a "good patient," that is, a submissive sufferer who fears empowerment, then you may as well close up shop. What we are trying to communicate to you is related to your potential. You are not a statistic. Survival mechanisms are built into you, but you must give your genes a live message if they are to respond. If you are open to sharing the mystical aspects of life rather than closing your mind and refusing to accept what you cannot understand, then read on. Yes, there are practical experiences, too, such as the advantages of humor and how to be empowered when interacting with health professionals.

Authority figures' words can kill or cure. When we are told that certain side effects will happen, they *can* indeed happen, even when we have been given a placebo. The mind is very powerful. We need to know that our thoughts and emotions create an internal environment, which needs to be related to healing and not to the complications of treatment. To quote

Joyce, "Adriamycin, by the way, is known as the red death." If that's what your mind believes, it can be, but if Adriamycin were seen as a gift from God, the side effects would not be a problem. She also talks about receiving ACT, short for Adriamycin, Cytoxan and Taxol. What if they called it CAT instead? I know of four chemotherapy drugs in a protocol that was called EPOH. One oncologist noted that if you turned the letters around, it became HOPE. He changed the name for his patients, and more of them responded to therapy. So rather than enter therapy in conflict, learn to visualize what you desire. Your thoughts and feelings need to be in unison, as Joyce demonstrates. The will to live is a real force, which affects everyone's life and health. When you draw a picture of your therapy as the devil giving you poison, you have a problem.

The message you live and transmit to your body is the issue. Survival behavior can be learned from the behavior portrayed by Joyce and Kevin and their families. They worked at healing their lives and bodies and, thus, did not empower their enemy, or disease. When you fight a war, you empower your enemy because that is what you focus on. The kill approach does not enhance your immune function or life, and then death becomes a failure on your part and you are a loser. When your focus is related to healing your life and body, you are a winner and have much to teach others about living, rather than about merely avoiding dying. Some people will do everything they "think" is the right thing, like being a vegetarian, meditating, and exercising, and they die anyway. The tragedy is, they were so busy doing all the "right" things, they forgot to *enjoy life*!

Joyce shares some very meaningful wisdom: "This is my lesson to share: Be happy with what you have right now. If you put your arms up and ask for what you need, you'll get it. Well, I was about to be hit with that brick I'd prayed for." Joseph Campbell writes that we need to love our fate and, no matter what hell happens, accept that it is what we need. When we are capable of that, it shifts our thinking. We learn from our wounds, and the despair and darkness, like charcoal under pressure, becomes a diamond. It is no longer "Why me?" but "Try me." You realize that your disease is not God punishing you but that it is a loss of your health. When you lose something, you go searching for what you have lost, as Joyce and Kevin had the courage to do. They were not focused on not dying, but on *living*, and the traditional and alternative choices that made sense to them. They decided which prescriptions to fill.

Their motivation led them to travel to Switzerland and have the courage and energy to do so. They reached out to family and friends for help and support, emotionally and financially. That is survival behavior. Others have the right to say no to what you ask for, but you have to have the courage to ask for help—and survivors do that. When they join a support group, it is a group that truly supports them and their efforts. It is not a group of victims who spend their time whining and complaining and, if they do not do well, blaming themselves for doing it wrong.

Joyce shares the concept of getting people to pay attention to their feelings when choosing what path in life to follow. I ask people, "What would you do if you had fifteen minutes to live?" The answer that taught me the most came from one of our sons: "I'd buy a quart of chocolate ice cream and eat it." So no matter what your answer is, ask yourself if it is your chocolate ice cream. If not, then change your answer and your life, and be born again.

Women live longer than men with the same cancers, and married men live longer than single men. Our lives are about our connections and relationships and meaning. Studies show that even pets are therapeutic. But it is important that we not live a role. Joyce's life should mean more than her being a mother, and Kevin should not simply be the wage earner. Why? Because I know women whose cancers recurred and they died when their kids left home, and men whose lives ended once they couldn't work anymore. I want you to live your authentic, meaningful life and relate to the world through your unlimited and unconditional love for yourself and others.

What happens when you live that way? I have many stories I can share about people who did not deny the likelihood of their impending death but went home to live until they died. That is what has kept me counseling and coaching people for over thirty years. One letter I received ended with "I didn't die, and now I'm so busy I'm killing myself. Help! Where do I go from here?" I told her to take a nap. And what about my landscaper friend John, age seventy? When I operated upon him, he just wanted to go home and make the world beautiful before he died. He refused treatment and died at age 94 with no sign of cancer.

There are no guarantees, but if you have self-worth and self-esteem and were brought up with love, you understand what I'm saying. Do not fear participating and giving it your best shot. If you grew up with indifference, rejection, and abuse, let my words and Joyce's book convince you that you are loved and worth the effort. False hope is an oxymoron. There can be false expectations, but hope is real. It's not about statistics; hope is necessary for survival.

It is a spiritual journey and not just a physical one. I love getting the wisdom I learn from country western music:

There are times in life when you gotta crawl,
Lose your grip and stumble and fall.
When you can't lean on no one else,
That's when you find yourself.

The going's easy when the road is flat.
Them danged hills will get you every time.
That's when you learn how to climb.

So to find your true self, learn how to climb, explore ways to heal your life, and give your body a LIVE message, read on.

Bernie Siegel, MD
Retired general/pediatric surgeon,
now involved in humanizing medical care and medical education.
Founder of Exceptional Cancer Patients (ECaP).
Author of numerous books, including *Love, Medicine & Miracles,*
Prescriptions for Living, Help Me to Heal, 365 Prescriptions for the Soul, and
Faith, Hope & Healing.
Academic codirector of the Experiential Health
and Healing Program at the Graduate Institute

TABLE OF CONTENTS

INTRODUCTION

My Dear Reader,

With tremendous gratitude, I thank you for sharing your precious time with me. Most likely, you have been guided to this book. You may have picked it up because our story intrigued you or because you're interested in improving your health. Perhaps you have an illness or ailment and have been told you must live with it for the rest of your life. You may have reached an overwhelming point of frustration physically, emotionally, or spiritually and are searching for a better way to live. Or, best of all, you may be healthy and want to remain healthy. Whatever the reason, the admiration I feel for your willingness to find a solution fills my heart.

I'll share my reasons for being so grateful. I have been given a gift—a gift that has prompted me to write this book. Ten years ago I was asleep, unconscious. Then my eyes were opened to a world I had never known existed.

In the past several years, I've gained knowledge and life experience that is more precious to me than the Hope Diamond. This knowledge is more valuable than anything I learned in eighteen years on Wall Street or during my grade school, high school, and college years combined. It's more valuable than any jewel because it is the most precious gift of all: the gift of life.

This gift includes the keys to an even better quality of life—a life that is healthy physically, emotionally, and spiritually. I've been given this gift and cannot possibly keep it to myself. It was meant to be shared, and I'm passionate about sharing it. I believe I have been given this precious gift because I was meant to share it with *you*.

I have discovered what I feel are secrets to modern-day health issues. I call them "secrets," not because they've been deliberately hidden, like the DaVinci Code, but because they remain largely undiscovered by the masses. Our discovery of these secrets and living them is the reason my husband and I are alive.

Although this is not intended as a "how-to," I have woven some of the secrets into my story and have validated them through the success of our healing. I have put the knowledge I've gained into practice in my own life and the lives of my family. As you might guess, I am passionate about sharing this information with anyone who is ready to hear it because of the dramatic, irrevocable, and transforming effect it had on me—which includes giving me the gift of life.

Perhaps you, too, will feel the hope, freedom, excitement, and exhilaration of knowing you can empower yourself to create results that lead to higher-quality, lasting health. Certain events in my life led me to this spectacular shift—a transformation that can't possibly be conveyed unless you know the details of my story.

* * *

My life was going great. Well, all right, maybe not *great,* but pretty good for a thirty-year-old kid from Queens, New York. My fourteen-year career on Wall Street was progressing rapidly, and I was managing the operations of a $2 billion business. My husband, Kevin, and I were building a dream house, which we planned to fill with a swarm of children—at least five. I swam; I skied; I attended night school and was learning to golf. Since I come from a family of golfers, I had dreams of becoming the next "Jack-lyn" Nicklaus.

Well, maybe not. I would have been happy just to get the ball off the ground and flying straight. I wasn't exactly good. My dad, a retired New York City police officer, had been semipro, and my mom, a retired Designer Department sales person for A&S Department Stores, had recently begun winning local golf tournaments, so why not me?

I had always wanted to experience life to the fullest. If there was something new and interesting or challenging to explore, I was all for it. Except, maybe, skydiving or cliff diving—I wasn't ready for that yet, but then, you never know…

Kevin was active, too. He played softball on a couple of teams, golfed, worked out, and had just started a new career. He'd moved from being a systems programmer at IBM to building power plants. *What?* A computer geek building power plants?

Doesn't matter. We were working hard, traveling with our friends, and having fun. As far as we knew, we were both healthy. I was even in my ideal weight zone! We were your typical thirtyish couple with no kids. Everything was cool. Our careers and living life to the fullest were where we were at, baby.

Or so we thought. One fateful day, that all changed. On a gorgeous spring day with not a cloud in the sky, my perfectly healthy husband had a brain hemorrhage, and three strokes—and we're not talking golf. These strokes left him paralyzed on his right side. Miraculously, he survived, but he needed brain surgery, and he went through the most horrific physical therapy imaginable. He was only thirty-one.

A year later, I was pregnant with our first baby—not all of Kevin was paralyzed! —but the doctors thought the baby had spina bifida. They wanted us to abort. We didn't.

When my baby was eight months old, I was diagnosed with stage 2b breast cancer. I was also given the devastating news that I couldn't have any more children. I was only thirty-three.

I lost my job on Wall Street. Along with my income, I also lost my medical insurance, disability insurance, and life insurance, and we were pretty close to losing our house, too.

A year later almost to the day, Kevin was diagnosed with stage 3b malignant melanoma. The cancer had already traveled to the lymph nodes in his groin, and suspicious spots were also evident on his lung, his shin, and a bone in his ankle. He was given a 20 to 30 percent chance of survival. He was thirty-four.

To top it all off with whipped cream, chocolate syrup, and a cherry, while my husband was still recovering from his treatments, we discovered that my oncologist and surgeon had misdiagnosed me. All that year, they had repeatedly told me not to worry, I was fine. By the time I convinced them things weren't fine, the cancer had reached stage 4. There is no stage 5. I was told that nothing could be done to save my life. I was thirty-five years old.

It didn't all happen in a week, but it sure felt like it. I guess we weren't as healthy as we thought! Our lives collapsed around us, but again and again we emerged from the rubble. Little by little, we repaired, rebuilt, and recreated our beliefs, our strength, our emotions, our lives, and our dreams.

All right, so life wasn't perfect and things were pretty stressful. But I have always held the belief that a ray of sunlight shines in any situation. You might get drenched trying to find it, but remember, the sun is always shining—it just might be behind the clouds." Our ray of sunlight is that ten years later, Kevin is walking, our child is perfectly healthy, and both Kevin and I are alive, well, and cancer free. Life has never been better. More than that, life is amazing!

With little hope available to us through conventional medicine, we took control of our health and journeyed into a world we hadn't known existed. The world of alternative medicine was one I knew little about—and certainly didn't have any faith in. But as we regained our health, I quickly became a believer.

This book will take you on our journey into a world of alternative options to conventional treatments. Our journey included European biological medicine, which identifies the root causes of why we get sick. You'll also learn about the benefits of the primarily raw, green, enzyme-rich, low-sugar diet that we used to strengthen and heal our bodies. The journey explores the physical, emotional, and spiritual aspects of healing. Our voyage of trust and faith led us to a clinic in the Swiss Alps. We also made a pilgrimage to a miraculous, mystical healing high atop a mountain in Italy.

Along the way, we learned not to focus on the quick fixes offered by toxic prescriptions that eliminate symptoms while masking the illness and causing side effects. Instead, we focused on removing the root causes of the illnesses and on building our bodies back up. This little-known world relies on cutting-edge diagnostics and treatments that include high-temperature heat therapy, detoxing, and immune system stimulation. I'll also identify some sneaky physical culprits that weaken us and that are tied to degenerative diseases. My purpose in sharing our journey is not to drag you into the cavernous misery of those insane years. My purpose is to provide information that will help you create a springboard for new hope—hope that inspires action. Hope that will draw you toward creating a better world, one where you can experience less ill-health and feel good … even great!

By making health our priority, we open ourselves to the possibility of having wonderful, vibrant lives. My purpose is to share our experience so that you, too, can benefit from the secrets we have learned.

My hope is that no one else has to experience the misery we did. Let's face it; you wouldn't wish that on your worst enemy. That's it in a nutshell: hope. More than anything, I hope you will say, "Wow, this is shocking! If it could happen to them at such a young age, it could happen to anyone … including me or my children. I really do need to take good care of myself and my family." And then take action!

It is my direct experience that many illnesses, including cancer, are preventable or reversible. So why not just prevent it? After all, it's much easier to prevent an illness than to reverse one—no ifs, ands, or buts. And, boy, have I spouted my share of ifs, ands, and buts! You might not agree with me, and you obviously don't have to. I understand—there's a tremendous amount of skepticism out there. I was one of the skeptics myself until I personally experienced the amazing improvement in my husband's and my health.

So with that, I invite you to laugh, cry, or maybe just smile. If you are drawn down, I pray you will then be raised back up, as we have been. Or you may just allow yourself to receive whatever you are meant to receive by reading our story.

I pray that you allow the power you hold within yourself to find the best way for you to heal any aspect of your life. I pray that you open yourself even to possibilities we might never be able to comprehend, and that you don't let that mystery stop you from achieving your dreams and health.

I wish for you a life filled with an abundance of blessings, good health, loving relationships, kindness, joy, and laughter. Welcome to my passion.

With love and warmest admiration for you and the power within you,

Joyce

Chapter One

IT'S GETTING CLOUDY:
BRAIN HEMORRHAGE

Where did it all begin? Oh, yeah, that's right: life was great.

Kevin was a boilermaker. Not the drink, but the guy who builds huge power plants. I was working my tush off and had just gotten promoted to senior vice president of an investment firm in Manhattan's financial district. No kids yet. We lived in Queens, in the home where I grew up. My parents lived in Florida, so we were living in their house while our dream home was going up on Long Island.

The avalanche began on March 1, 1996. It was a gorgeous spring morning, not a cloud in the sky, and I left for work around six, as usual. Your typical Wall Street workaholic, I wanted to get some work done in the calm before the craziness hit.

Then I got the call. It took me a moment to recognize the slurred voice. It was Kevin—thirty-one and healthy as a horse. Out with coworkers last night for a meeting and a few drinks, he got in a little late and slept on the couch so he wouldn't wake me. He sounded tired and hungover.

"I feel a little funny," he slurred. "Think I pinched a nerve or something— I'm a little numb down my arm and leg."

I would soon see how much Kevin downplayed things. Seems he'd gone up to the bedroom after I left, then woke up feeling funny.

"Okay," I said. "Let me call my parents and I'll call you back."

7

I mean, what else do you do when you don't know what else to do? Don't parents know everything? That's part of their job, right? (Unless, of course, you're between the ages of twelve and twenty—but after that, it's amazing how much they learn.) My parents said we should call the doctor—a logical suggestion, especially since they were 1,500 miles away. So I called Kevin back and set up a conference call with our doctor. He confirmed the likelihood of a pinched nerve but said call back if it wasn't better in fifteen minutes.

I went back to work, figuring it would unkink on its own. But fifteen minutes later, Kevin called again to say it wasn't better. Nothing could have prepared me for the magnitude of what was to come.

His doctor said, "He might have a pinched nerve or maybe a TIA." Wait—wasn't TIA when your jaw was out of whack and you had to wear one of those mouth thingies while you slept?

The doc said, "Since it hasn't gotten better and he's having trouble walking, you might want to call an ambulance."

What! An ambulance? *It's a pinched nerve,* I thought. No one was raising any alarms. Nothing was registering. I asked, "What's a TIA?"

"It's like a mini stroke."

This definitely wasn't registering. My mind raced. Kevin was way too young and fit for a stroke, mini or any other kind. In my bewilderment, childhood memories flooded over me. My grandmother had suffered a stroke. It paralyzed her, and she could never speak another word. She lived with us and just made these catlike sounds and grunts and groans and had to have a portable toilet next to her bed.

That didn't sound at all like what was going on with Kevin. Kevin could talk. It *must* just be a pinched nerve—the very idea of a "mini stroke" was absurd. He couldn't actually be talking to me and not be basically okay.

But I didn't yet realize how Kevin downplayed everything. "A little numb" meant *he was paralyzed!*

Since I didn't know he was paralyzed, my mind was on mundane thoughts of how to get back home, which was at least an hour away. I would have to order a car to get from Manhattan to Queens.

"I don't want you to call the ambulance until you're closer," Kevin said.

"Why?"

"I'd rather you were here. I don't want the ambulance to come and all the neighbors to see me leave the house like that. I want you to be here."

I thought I understood his embarrassment. After all, didn't you have to be bleeding or unconscious before doing anything as extreme as calling an ambulance? Still, this was my *husband.*

"I don't think we should wait," I said. "I should call them now."

Then he switched to his stern, I've-made-my-decision-and-don't-piss-me-off voice. "No. I don't want you to call the ambulance until you're almost here."

I was naive. Besides, when he used that voice, everything was final.

I had the car company send someone right away. I stayed calm because this was all still just "a little numb" and "feeling a little funny" and "a pinched nerve"—nothing more.

Once I got into the car, my head began swirling. I called for the ambulance when I was fifteen minutes away. I arrived just as the ambulance did. What a scary sight! The flashing lights reflected off the brick row houses. When I was a kid, one of the older neighbors had been taken away in an ambulance. He never came back.

Inside my head, a little voice said, *Excuse me, but do we really need all this attention? It's a bit much for a pinched nerve, don't you think?* Then that feeling of sickness came over me. It *was* just a pinched nerve, right?

I unlocked the door for the paramedics, and we all walked in together.

"Where is he, ma'am?" one of the paramedics asked.

Excuse me, aren't I a little young to be called "ma'am"? "He's upstairs," I said.

They asked me to wait downstairs so I wouldn't be in their way. In retrospect, I realize that since they didn't know what they were going to find, they didn't need to deal with me if I freaked out. But I'm not a freak-out kind of person—not until after the immediate emergency is over, anyway.

Those few minutes seemed an eternity. When they finally let me come upstairs, Kevin was already being strapped into a stretcher, which had been propped up so he could sit upright. Big orange straps pinned his arms so the EMTs could navigate the stairs more easily.

"What do you think is wrong?" I asked.

"We aren't sure," one said. "He might have had a TIA."

That word again. My face looked as if I'd just bitten down on a sour cherry. Kevin looked a little scared. It was awful to see my strong, healthy husband in that stretcher, but he managed to joke with the guys.

The paramedics carried all 190 pounds of him plus the stretcher down those narrow stairs. After that, they still had to manage the front stoop. My next-door neighbor was just coming home. The look of shock on her face really stood out. I must have looked just as shocked and terrified, like a deer in headlights.

"What's wrong?" she asked.

The word "mini-stroke" came out of my mouth. Then reality hit. I gagged as tears welled up and I began shaking. But I couldn't let my husband see how scared I was, so I blinked back the tears and acted calm and in control.

They took him to the hospital. I think I drove myself there—I actually don't remember, but since my car was in the lot, I must have. When I arrived, the nurses wouldn't let me in.

"They're getting him settled in," one explained. "You'll have to wait."

Wait? I didn't want to wait. I wanted to know what was going on! The agony began as I watched every minute on the clock crawl by. My best friend, Diane, worked at the hospital and met me there.

"It's probably nothing," she said, but she looked more scared than I did. Since she was very intuitive, that freaked me out.

I waited and waited, but they still wouldn't let me see him. Finally, the doctor came out.

"We need to run some scans," he said. "We need to see if he's bleeding in the brain."

What? Another sour-cherry look. Bleeding in the brain? But he was only thirty-one.

What seemed like hours later, they finally let me see him, but only for a minute. He was clearly scared. I tried to remain optimistic, but I was terrified. They shooed me out until they were ready to do the scans.

They let me go with him through the endless maze of corridors and down to the basement, where a different doctor asked the same questions I had already heard half a dozen times: "Did you have any headaches recently? Any dizziness or numbness?"

Nope, nope, and nope

Then he asked a new one. "Do you smoke?"

"Um, yes," Kevin said.

"No," I chimed indignantly, "he doesn't smoke."

"Do you smoke?" the doctor asked Kevin again.

"Yes.

"How much?" the doctor asked.

"About a pack a day," Kevin answered, trying not to look at me.

"No, he doesn't." I was very firm. I was, after all, the knowing, informed, caring wife. "He's just confused because of the brain bleeding."

Diane gently put her hand on my arm. "Joyce," she said, "I think you should let him answer."

I assumed Kevin didn't know what he was talking about. After all, smoking had been a big factor in our marriage. The night we first met, I had walked into a local bar and restaurant. Although the place was packed, I spotted him right away. He was a little way down the bar; wearing a bright blue button-down shirt that highlighted the brightest blue eyes I'd ever seen.

Wow! And he was staring at me! I had the urge to turn around and look behind me to see who he was looking at. I felt a little awkward, but he didn't take his eyes off me as I walked past. My friend Suzanne, whom I hadn't seen in a couple of years, had called me out of the blue and we decided to go out that night. It must be destiny when a friend suddenly reappears and, next thing you know, you're out on a Saturday night and spot a really cute guy!

As Suzanne and I talked and caught up, I glanced back at him a few times, remaining cool. Each time I looked back, he turned toward me and smiled. I had that feeling of butterflies. Then he took out a cigarette.

My father was a three-pack-a-day smoker. Smoke literally gave me a headache and made me feel nauseated. Aside from that, I just couldn't stand the smell.

As Kevin lit up, I dropped my sweet smile and shot him a look of disgust. He instantly broke the cigarette in half, dropped it, and stomped it out. When I laughed, he came over. The rest is history. Kevin quit smoking. We got engaged the next year and were married a year after that.

We'd been together eight years. He had always said he didn't smoke anymore, so I got the eight-year-old news flash there in the hospital.

The doctor, meanwhile, shook his head. He couldn't understand how a healthy thirty-one-year-old could be free of any aneurism symptoms yet bleeding in his brain. They ran endless hours of testing. The angiogram was very painful. A catheter holding a tiny camera was threaded into a vein in his groin and run way up inside his body.

Diane finally left to return to work. We waited. Then the awful news came: it wasn't a TIA. That would have been the better scenario. Instead, Kevin had an AVM: an arteriovenous malformation. An AVM is similar to a brain aneurism in that they both involve bleeding in the brain. Kevin had a brain hemorrhage. He also had suffered *three* strokes. He would need brain surgery. He would be admitted to intensive care immediately. If the bleeding didn't stop on its own, he might not survive the night.

Kevin remained extremely calm. He did have that *Oh, shit* look, though. He reminded me of a scared little boy putting on a good front. He was as sweet as could be, trying to joke with everyone to make them more at ease— until a guy tried to put an A-line (a small plastic catheter) into the artery in his left arm … and tried, and tried.

Kevin hated the guy and let him know it. Sticking a tube into a vein is not the easiest thing to do, and it's supposed to be done by highly trained personnel. This guy was new at it. So were we, for that matter. At one point, he climbed on top of the bed and straddled Kevin. Although my husband handles pain well and doesn't usually complain, he finally screamed, then told the guy to get someone who knew what they were doing.

It had been a really long day. The ordeal had started around seven in the morning, and it was now six p.m. I maintained my calm exterior, but inside, the anxiety was spinning out of control. My stomach and head felt it the most, while my heart pounded like a jackhammer. Maybe they should be running some tests on me while they were at it. My heart wasn't supposed to be doing this.

As we went to intensive care, family and friends had already started to arrive. Thank God for them. The support was a real godsend. Kevin's brothers, my brother and sister, our friends, and his mother came. His sister Patty was already on her way in from Michigan, and my mom was making arrangements to fly up from Florida. Even my assistant showed up, toting my Rolodex. At least twenty people milled around outside the ICU. Prayer chains were started as those who could handle it were granted a couple of minutes to see him, knowing that it might be the last time.

Seeing everyone was a nice distraction. It helped keep me from thinking of the horrible alternatives: Would he survive the night? Survive the surgery? Would he ever feed himself again? Ever walk again?

That was one of the longest days and nights of my life. The others were yet to come.

After a time, visiting hours were over, and the family left. I couldn't leave—didn't want to leave. How could I, knowing he might not make it through the night? The nurses were so kind, they didn't force me to go home. I fought sleep, and when I caught myself falling off, I quickly opened my eyes, tuning in to make sure all the machines were beeping along at their usual rhythm.

Thankfully, Kevin was still alive in the morning—the first thing to be grateful for. The next afternoon, my mom arrived. Everything felt better once she came. I always called her "Mom," not "Mommy," but that's how I felt: like a little girl who needed her mommy. There's no replacement for a mother's hug when you're terrified.

Once our family returned that afternoon, the nurses assured me I could make a quick trip to the house. Besides, Kevin wanted me to take a break. I wanted to pack some things to bring back for him. I also needed to get cleaned up and change my clothes—after two days in the hospital, I was pretty skanky. I hadn't even brushed my teeth.

I was also still maintaining control as best I could. I was afraid to cry, as if crying would confirm that it all was actually happening. But then I walked into the darkened house and went upstairs. In our room, I saw the mess that had been left behind. The comforter and sheets had been pulled off the bed; the phone was on the floor; the smell of urine from when Kevin couldn't make it to the bathroom hung in the air; the things from the night table had been knocked over.

That's when it hit me, when the enormity of what had happened became real: his struggle, his pain, his sheer panic. I broke down. Racking sobs shook me until I fell to my knees. Oh, dear God, the poor guy! He went through such hell. He must have been so terrified lying there on the floor. And even then he had made me wait to call the ambulance. He could have died right here!

He still could die.

"Oh, dear God," I prayed, "please let him be okay."

Feeling physically, mentally, and emotionally drained and fearful of what was to come, I dragged myself over to the tissue box and sat on the bed, pulling out tissue after tissue and sobbing uncontrollably.

Then something unimaginable happened. I'd never experienced anything like it before and never have since. Yet there was no doubt: someone sat on the bed next to me. Not a flesh-and-blood person, but a being. I actually felt the bed sag under its weight. Something touched my shoulders, as if I were being comforted.

For a split second there was another kind of fear—that "scary movie" feeling. I was alone in a big, dark house. Immediately behind that, a sense of peace came over me. It was Kevin's father, who had passed away a few years earlier. I was certain of it. He was telling me he was here and that Kevin was going to be fine.

I realized that there was a much more powerful force out there than anything we can comprehend. About the most uncanny thing that had ever happened to me before was having streetlights black out when I passed them in the car or walked under them. I never really paid much attention to that, though. This was far more powerful.

* * *

Back at the hospital, I quickly fell into what would be my routine for the next month. Since the bleeding in Kevin's brain had slowed, the doctors wanted to wait four weeks to do the surgery, hoping to improve the chances of regaining some movement. Since performing the surgery immediately could cause further permanent paralysis, waiting was actually safer.

For the next month, I went between work and the hospital every day. It was agonizing to watch Kevin. He began physical therapy in the hospital, but nothing was happening. When he was finally released, he started an intense physical therapy regimen. He should have gone into an inpatient treatment center, but he just wanted to go home. This was another one of those times when there was just no convincing him.

Eventually, he regained some movement in his right arm and was able to use it more. His right side, though, was completely paralyzed from the waist down. Dead. Nothing. *Nada.* Zippo. So the physical therapy tried to teach his brain how to tell his leg to move again. Neither was in the mood to cooperate. The determination he exerted would have moved a building, but nothing happened. It was torture to see this strong man grunting and groaning and turning purple, veins popping out on his forehead, yet unable to move one toe.

By this time, my mom had pretty much moved back from Florida. To this day, I thank God she was there. She took care of Kevin so I could work. I don't know how I would have been able to do it without her. The people at work—my partners and the president as well as my staff—gave me such great support. Because of them, I was able to work the early part of the day and then come home for the late afternoon to care for Kevin.

Every day, a handicap van took Kevin to physical therapy. He was going through so much just to be able to walk again. He was so determined, he would lean on a walker and use his upper body to swing the leg around.

I'll never forget the first time he moved his big toe. It was as though a miracle had happened—no, it *was* a miracle.

That was the defining moment. The moment of hope. Up until that point, we hadn't known if he would ever walk again. Now at least we had hope. No guarantees, of course, but hope. How beautiful a toe can be, and what an utter miracle that we can wiggle them!

Even more amazing was the day he first took a step. We drove down to a lake near our house, and he shuffled along with his walker. At one point, the path narrowed, so I took the lead.

"Hey, Joyce," he said, "look!"

I turned. He hoisted the walker off the ground and took a single tiny step. He was clumsy, and the walker slapped back down, but it was as if he had just walked on the moon! The look on his face was priceless. He had such a boyish grin and was so excited. I'll never forget that day. He had a long way to go, and it still didn't mean he would ever walk on his own, but it sure was a good sign.

The surgery was terrifying. After hours of torturous waiting—hours of not knowing whether he would make it—I was allowed to see him. Seeing someone after brain surgery is pretty gruesome. Kevin looked like a mummy, with tubes full of blood coming out of his skull. I'm a strong person, but it did me in—I fainted.

In the end, it was successful. They were able to repair the AVM and put in a metal plate. Now he just has a hole in his head. Well, it's more like a gully actually, so we hope he never goes bald. And we're a little nervous walking through metal detectors at the airport.

During the course of many months of intense physical therapy, Kevin regained about 90 percent of the movement in his right leg. It's still obvious that he has to consciously tell his leg to move, and the foot sort of flops down. Even though his construction job takes him 180 feet up in the air across skinny beams, he went back to work. No one thought he would be able to return to his job, but Kevin would not give up.

He still works hard at walking. The effect becomes very noticeable when he's tired or has had a drink. He also has difficulty running, walking fast, taking the stairs, and walking in loafers. But given that his "pinched nerve" could easily have killed or permanently paralyzed him, he's truly a walking miracle.

This was the first of several miracles. There was no mistaking that divine intervention, combined with the power of prayer and personal determination, made all the difference. We have many angels that look over us, surround us, and offer guidance and comfort.

Some things we still laugh about. When Kevin tried to feed himself, I would watch him try to get the spoon near his mouth. It would have been so much easier for me to feed him, but, of course, I wasn't allowed—by the doctors or by him. Turns out that watching him was much more fun. All I could think about was feeding a baby and zooming the spoon around like an airplane. Kevin did the same thing, getting it near his mouth without necessarily getting it inside.

They say laughter is the best medicine. . . .

Chapter Two

IT'S RAINING: SPINA BIFIDA

Things were getting back to normal. Kevin was back to work and making adjustments to compensate for the loss of movement in his leg. Oh, did I mention that during his AVM, we were having a house built forty-five minutes from my parents' home? So there were all kinds of decisions and paperwork and similar things that demanded our attention.

And the builders were not the nicest people. In fact, they were pretty cold and heartless during Kevin's hospitalization. During that first month, they told us we would lose the house and the down payment if we didn't make our selections and come up with more money. Countertops, cabinets, and flooring were the furthest things from our minds. This was not the easiest thing, what with the medical bills, Kevin's being unable to work—possibly *never* being able to work again—and the lack of sleep.

It all worked out, and eight months after Kevin's episode, we moved into our dream home. No furniture to speak of, other than my parents' twenty-year-old hand-me-downs, but four beautiful walls, and a lot of dirt around the outside. Since life is short, we decided not to wait any longer to start a family. I got pregnant with our first child.

During this time, my company was being bought out, so things were a little stressful at work, with a lot of demands that had to be met as we prepared for the buyout.

But I was thrilled with my pregnancy. I don't think I'd ever been so excited in all my life. I just loved the feeling of having a little person growing inside me. I just knew it was going to be someone amazing. We were excited, but I waited patiently for the traditional three months to pass before telling anyone.

Then the next little hurdle appeared. Did I say "little hurdle"? It was more like the Berlin Wall. During some routine testing, I heard the shocking news: the doctors believed our baby had spina bifida, and wanted us to consider aborting.

From my nonmedical perspective, I would describe spina bifida as an incompletely formed spinal column. The spinal cord can protrude through the opening in the bones, leaving it open and vulnerable to damage. Anencephaly—the absence of a major portion of the brain and skull—was also possible.

Talk about a punch in the gut. I went from being a deliriously happy expectant mother to a terrified person facing the decision whether to take a life. I pray to God that no one else ever has to make the same decision. This was a whole different category of stress—floating on air one second, completely distraught the next.

I continued keeping silent about the pregnancy in case the baby didn't survive. My stomach got bigger and bigger … and bigger! I tried to keep wearing the same suits to make the changes less obvious. I used lots of safety pins to hold my zippers together.

I wasn't fooling anyone. Come on! I probably ate twice as much and really started to pack on the pounds. No, I was not one of those graceful pregnant women with a tight basketball for a tummy. Instead, I had several basketballs: one in my stomach, one on my left hip, one my right hip, and two soccer balls on my chest. I could have been a Harlem Globetrotter, hanging onto all those balls!

Then came test after test after test. This doctor's visit, that counseling session, another test. I was beginning to have a real aversion to hospitals. By my fifth month, people were beginning to ask questions. We had to choose.

It didn't matter whether our child had spina bifida. God had given this child to us, and we would deal with whatever came our way. We started telling people I was pregnant. I continued to feel good—really, really good. I just loved having that baby in my belly. I was certain it was a boy. We could even see his little peeshie on the sonogram, and being the expert sonographers that all expectant parents assume themselves to be, we just knew it was a boy. Although I had that nagging concern about my child's health, things seemed to be progressing as expected.

Work was so crazy, I didn't have any time to spend preparing to have the baby—I was too busy preparing to be away from work and to work from home. I didn't even give my mother the registry list early enough. The shower was scheduled early, but I really wasn't prepared. The baby's room wasn't even done.

We did make it to one Lamaze class. The first day was really cool. We were uptight, so we made some jokes—you know, the "I'm nervous so I'll laugh, but I'm really trying to act cool, but, oh, no, is this really happening?" kind of jokes. We laughed a lot. Besides, everybody else had already done this, so we figured they'd tell us what to do when we got to the hospital.

We didn't really pay close attention. We figured the instructors would give us a summary at the last class. I still had lots to get done. We didn't do all that last-month stuff like buying diapers and baby wipes, or setting up a changing table and a baby bath. There was still that hesitation, that nervousness, the superstition and the what-ifs.

That first Lamaze class came at the beginning of my eight month. The next day, I had my first internal exam. I was running late because we had scheduled the first big meeting with the buyers of our company for the next morning. It was also the beginning of the month, so we were finishing up last month's deal closings.

I felt great, though. I was so excited—our first internal! The doctor would give me a much better idea of how the baby was doing, if it was dropping into position, and an overall "How ya doin' down there?"

So he begins the exam. All talking and laughing, then he probes a little more. A little less laughing, and he probes some more.

It's really starting to hurt. No more laughing. Now I'm getting nervous. He's really digging in. I think his whole fist is gone. *Jeez, doc, can you take it a little easier?*

It all rushed over me. *Oh, no, what's wrong? It's the spina bifida.* The baby wasn't responding. Thinking back, it hadn't moved in the past several days. It was usually really active—so active it never slept. I was panic-stricken. Deer-in-the-headlights time again. *Oh, my God, the baby's dead!* A hiccup of a sob escaped me.

"What's wrong?" I managed.

He popped his head up and ripped off his gloves. "Nothing. Everything's great."

"Are you kidding me?"

"This baby isn't coming anytime soon. You still have lots of time. Your due date should be around October sixth—at least a month away."

I was dumbfounded. Was he joking? He just about gave me a heart attack! After all the time he spent down there, I was *sure* something was wrong. *Jeez Louise, Doc.* And off he bounced to his next patient, leaving me to catch my breath. Well, at least the pregnancy was moving along the way it should.

Several hours later, around 2 a.m., I woke up feeling really weird. As the pregnancy progressed, I was forever getting up at night to pee. I must have been having one of those dreams where I thought I was peeing. Normally I didn't lose it, but all kinds of crazy things happen when you're pregnant. So I woke up, and, oh, my God! I really *had* peed during my dream.

How embarrassing! But that's pregnancy for you. I went to the bathroom, changed my wet clothes, and went back to bed. Then I woke up a second time. I peed in my dream again! What the heck? Why couldn't I control that? It just came out without my even realizing it.

I went to the bathroom and put a pad and some towels on. I had to get up in a few hours to get ready for the meeting, and this was getting ridiculous. It couldn't be that my water broke—the doctor said I still had a lot more time. Something wasn't right, but I felt stupid calling the doctor at three a.m. to ask such a ridiculous question.

About an hour later, I decided I should ask Kevin what he thought. I felt bad waking him up, because he had to get up early, too. I woke him up anyway.

"Honey," I said, "you remember what they said at the first Lamaze class about the water breaking? Was there supposed to be a plug or something?"

"Huh? Whah …? I don't know …"

Snore—right back to sleep. The question hadn't even fazed him. I guess I should have started with some simpler questions like, "What's your name? When's your birthday?" I had a better chance of getting an answer out of a rock.

So I changed the towels, stared at the ceiling, changed the towels again, stared at the ceiling some more. I was just trying to make it to a more decent hour when I could call the doctor and get this straightened out and go to the meeting. I couldn't count sheep any longer, so I just tapped my finger and figured my water couldn't have broken. No plug had come out, and I didn't have contractions. So what the heck was going on?

As I called the doctor's answering service, I felt unbelievably stupid. Someone rang right back. It was my gynecologist's cute partner, the doctor whom I hadn't really spent any quality time with yet. I explained what was going on.

"Are you having contractions?" he asked.

"No."

"You need to come right in."

"I can't. I have a big meeting this morning."

"You need to come right in. It sounds like your water broke."

"But it couldn't have. The doctor told me I had plenty of time."

"It sounds like your water broke and you're not having contractions. The baby could be in distress. You need to come right in."

"I'm soaking wet, Doc," I said. "Can I at least take a shower?"

"No. You're thirty minutes to an hour away, and it's rush hour. You need to get here right away."

I knew he was right—I needed to go in. But I was sure it was nothing.

Well, because I wasn't really prepared and still hadn't done the things on my last-month checklist, I didn't even have a hospital bag packed. Looking back, I see I was either in denial or just oblivious. Either way, I wasn't really ready to have this baby.

I'll just go get it checked out, I thought. *The baby will check out fine; then I'll come home, shower, and head in to the office.* I woke my husband and told him what was going on.

"Wow, you're kidding!" he said. "Why didn't you wake me?"

Oh, what a gift to be able to sleep through anything!

So we raced to the hospital. We took back roads, wondering if we would need a police escort. But the angels and the good Lord were with us that day, because we hit only one red light the whole way. Our doctor's partner, the very cute, very young guy, was there. I couldn't believe he was a doctor. As he ran all kinds of tests and did an internal exam, I joked, "Should you really be doing this on our first date, Doc? I mean, I hardly know you and you're getting awfully personal."

"Yup," he said, "your water broke."

God, I wish I'd paid better attention in that Lamaze class. But they probably hadn't even covered that part yet.

"Can you just stop it?" I asked. "I can come right back after work. Maybe by then the contractions will have begun."

"Unfortunately, you can't just stop it," he chuckled.

I hoped he wouldn't ask me if I'd bothered to attend Lamaze class.

"The baby isn't ready to come out yet," he said.

"Okay, great, so I'll just come back when it is."

"Nope. You'll have to stay. If the contractions don't start in a couple of hours, we'll have to induce labor. So long as the baby remains stable, we won't have to do an emergency C-section."

"This can't be happening. The doctor said I had plenty of time."

"When was that?"

"Last night."

"What did he do when he saw you?"

"I had my first internal."

Then the grin appeared. He'd just gotten one over on the older, more experienced partner. "He did an internal, huh?"

"Yes. He had to dig pretty deep, but he finally found the baby and said I had plenty of time."

"He did, did he?" Then he laughed. "He broke your water."

"What?"

"When he was probing, he broke your water with that hook finger of his." He chuckled as he curled his finger.

"You have got to be kidding me!" I hollered. "I need to talk to him. Now!"

I was a pissed, decidedly premature pregnant woman who was not at all prepared for any of this. I had way too much to do before the baby was born. I had lots to do at work, I didn't have a changing table set up—I didn't even have diapers yet!

The baby remained stable, thank God, and the contractions started and then stopped. So they began inducing, but no dice on the baby making an appearance. He was having fun playing hide-and-seek. I was about to spend the next thirty-six hours in labor. So they put me in a room, and some of my friends and family visited while we waited. It was like slow torture.

I spent the next twenty-four hours watching coverage of Princess Diana's funeral. There wasn't a single other thing on TV, and this was before portable DVD players. It was a horrible day. I was devastated by Diana's death, in labor, feeling about as miserable as one could feel, and just wanting to move things along. But there would be nothing of the sort. This baby was not ready, and it didn't care that it no longer had a big, warm bath to swim around in.

Well, none of that mattered—all that mattered was that the baby was healthy. But I really didn't want to wait forever to find out if it had spina bifida. They induced labor and gave me a crazy drug that made me hallucinate without doing a thing for the pain. About the worst high you could possibly imagine.

Still nothing. My parents flew up from Florida. My mom came in and out of the room while I was drugged. I asked the same question each time: "Hi, Mom. When did you get here?"

Now I really wanted to kill "the hook." No epidural, and I still wasn't dilating. He'd broken my water, and this chicken wasn't even close to cooked. I hadn't been ready last night, but by now I was past ready. I wanted the pain to stop, and "the hook" was nowhere to be found.

After thirty-six hours of excruciating labor, my beautiful child made its debut in this world—but wasn't breathing. After an eternity of panic on my part, they managed to get it breathing, and I nearly fainted from relief. A team of five specialists was called in to check the baby out since we had both the spina bifida issue and its being a premie. Two of them turned to us and gave a thumbs-up. Our perfectly healthy, perfectly normal (if a little jaundiced) five-pound daughter was here.

That's right. I said "daughter." That was the next shock. We didn't even have a name for a little girl. We had two for a little boy because we were certain we were having a boy. Being doctors, we had seen it on the sonogram, remember? We saw the peeshie.

Oh, who cared? She was alive and healthy and didn't have spina bifida! We welcomed Kelsey O'Brien into the world. I had to admit that she did look a lot like a scrawny, undercooked Perdue chicken. Which reminded me, I was really hungry. *Anybody got a Whopper?* I needed some sleep.

Chapter Three

IT'S POURING: STAGE 2B

Life was crazy. I had a newborn and a demanding job, and I decided to surprise my mom and dad by going down to Florida. They hadn't seen Kelsey in two months, and my mother was suffering major withdrawal. We showed up when she wasn't home, and waited. When the car pulled into the driveway, we put Kelsey in the carrier seat and left her at the door.

When Mom walked in, her expression was priceless. She couldn't put it together. She had no idea why there was a child in her doorway, and at first she didn't even recognize Kelsey, because it made no sense. She finally put it together and said laughingly "What are *you* doing here?"

That's when we popped out from behind the couch, yelling, "Surprise!" She was ecstatic.

We had just settled in and told her how we arranged the visit with Dad when I got a phone call. My two partners, whom I loved, were leaving the company. I needed to go back immediately.

The next couple of months were challenging, to say the least. I was promoted to managing director and running a very successful business inside the firm, where I was responsible for $2 billion in client assets. I really needed a vacation because I hadn't had one since all the stress began a year ago. Staying home when your child is born is about the most nonvacation type of leave there is. It's work!

We decided to visit Beaches Resort in Jamaica. Our little girl was eight months old and the cutest, funniest, sweetest little thing, with enormous cheeks. Those were the days when we beamed over the littlest things, like her sitting up by herself and eating Cheerios off the table one at a time, or squishing scrambled eggs through her fingers as she tried to get them in her mouth with those huge cheeks bulging like a squirrel's. My friend, Greg, joked with me, "How many chestnuts do you think she could store in those cheeks for winter?" They were so big, they jiggled when she chewed.

We had just settled in at the hotel, and I showered before we went out to dinner. I thought how great it was to be on vacation and to have this beautiful new baby with us. I was exhausted but happy. As the water poured over me, I remembered something from a Barbara Walters news story. It was rare that I could find time to watch television, so my guardian angels had been looking over me that day. Little did I know that Barbara's story would save my life.

The story was about a young mom, around my age, who had just had a baby and was on vacation when she discovered a lump in her breast. *Well,* I thought, *now's as good a time as any to do my own breast exam.* As I let the water help my fingers slide over my skin, I thought of Erin Kramp and how moving and sad her story had been. Her lump was malignant breast cancer that ultimately metastasized. She was in stage 4, the last stage, and knew she was going to die. But she came up with a way to be a part of her daughter's life even after she was gone.

She prepared a set of writings, mementos, and videotapes. On the recordings, she offered advice about boys and dating and how to respect herself. She created different gifts to be given to her daughter on her birthdays and for special occasions, including her wedding day. She even said it would be okay for her husband to remarry and that she wanted her daughter to have another mommy. What an incredible woman! And how sad that she had to leave! The show was so moving, I had cried. The tears welled up as I thought of how sad it was.

Standing there in the shower, I felt something odd in my breast. Hmm. I'd never noticed anything there before. Had I? I wasn't sure. I tried to convince myself this was nothing unusual. I felt it again. Yes, something was definitely there. Actually, it was huge.

Oh, no, it couldn't be … could it? And then that sinking feeling came again—a sort of foreboding. *Oh, God. What if it is?* Then I started crying, thinking of Erin Kramp and my beautiful, happy, sweet daughter playing in the next room.

Okay, that's enough, said the little voice in my head. *Pull yourself together. Whatever it is, you'll deal with it.* I got out and didn't even bother to dry my hair—just pulled it back into a ponytail, which I rarely wore.

When I came out of the bathroom, my husband took my picture. Oh, great. Now I had a picture of the moment I discovered my lump. I smiled anyway. Wasn't that what you were supposed to do for the camera, no matter how you felt? I told him what I'd found, and he said, "Don't worry. I'm sure it's nothing."

This from the man who had said he had a pinched nerve when his brain was bleeding. Now, that was comforting. *Ugh!* The bad part was that we were in Jamaica and it was only Saturday, the first day of our vacation. I had to wait until Monday even to call the doctor, then wait another week until we flew back to see him.

"Kevin, maybe we should leave," I said.

"Sure, honey," he said. "If you want to leave, we will."

He was always so supportive. Obviously, I didn't want to leave.

"Maybe we should just talk to the doctor first," he said. "Then, if he says to go, we can hop on the first plane back to New York."

Well, I thought, we might as well live it up in the meantime. I remember saying that to myself again and again. If this was my last vacation, I might as well do it right. We had a blast, even though that sinking feeling stuck around the whole time. Quite a few piña coladas later, we decided to go cliff diving. Yes, cliff diving. Kelsey stayed in the kids' camp, where she had a ball, and we took off for the cliffs.

Did I mention there was a booze cruise before the launch? Sure, why not? If I was going to die from cancer, I might as well be able to say I'd gone cliff diving. Wasn't that important? To be able to look back and say I'd done something great? In their last moments, doesn't everyone regret that they haven't gone cliff diving? Or skydiving? And if I was going to go cliff diving, there really should be alcohol involved, right? In fact, there had better be alcohol involved.

Sounded like a great plan—until I got to the top of the cliff. That was about the dumbest thing we'd ever done. The multiple piña coladas couldn't possibly have prepared me for when I looked down, but the return trip on foot would be even more treacherous. No way was I going to jump! But at least thirty strangers waiting in line behind me and down below agreed that I should. Sure, they had also had quite a few piña coladas, but no matter— they knew what they were talking about … didn't they?

I don't recommend this one. I reiterate, it was the single dumbest thing we had ever done. I will never do it again, even though it's fun to say, "I thought I might have cancer, so I went cliff diving." It was not one of those "Wow, that was a truly momentous experience" moments. It was more like "Wow, that was a god-awful dumb thing to do."

"Terrifying" was not the word. After about fifteen minutes of torturing myself, and with a lot of encouragement, I did it, because climbing back down looked equally dangerous. How could everyone else have made it look so easy? It wasn't. I hit the water like a brick and was stone-cold sober in a split second.

There had been no coaching, so Kevin's face hit the water first. I went in with my knees bent in a sitting position. He chipped a tooth, and I wound up with a black and blue and purple mark from my tailbone to the back of my knee. I couldn't sit down for a week. I think I bruised my tailbone as well. The black and blue also looked great in a bathing suit.

The rest of the trip was a little more subdued. On Monday, the doctor said he thought it was nothing. Lumps were common after pregnancy because the body changed so much, and it was very rare for someone my age to have cancer. But he told me to come in when we got back, so that we could check it out anyway.

*   *   *

We made it out of Jamaica alive, and I walked into the doctor's office the following Monday, still unable to sit comfortably. I was a little concerned but kept reassuring myself with the phrase "these lumps are common after pregnancy." Still, every imaginable thought ran through my head, until he gave me the good news.

"I don't think it's anything," he said, "but go and have a sonogram to be sure. Also, visit this surgeon. This happens a lot after pregnancy. I don't think it is anything to worry about." Did I mention this was the "the hook," the same doctor who broke my water prematurely after telling me I had nothing to worry about, that the baby wasn't coming anytime soon?

Life was good again! I bounced out of his office. I planned to check it out, of course, but *yah, mon, everything is cool runnings.* (All right, so maybe I brought a little too much Jamaica home with me.)

Mom had come up to help my sister-in-law, who had just given birth to my goddaughter. She stopped by to say hello. I told her the good news and asked if she wanted to feel the lump. After all, wouldn't anybody? So I lay down on the bed and directed.

"See?" I said. "I actually think there are two lumps: a small one and a really large one. When I try to move one, it kind of pushes the other out of the way."

She agreed that it felt like two lumps. Two tumors don't usually appear next to each other, right? Of course not. So I booked the appointments in the first available time slots for later in the week. The sonogram would be followed by the surgeon's appointment.

I went for the sonogram by myself. That was a huge mistake. They came in; they went out; they came in; they went out; then another doctor came in. They went out; another came in. Are you getting the picture that maybe something's not quite right? My expectations that everything was fine dwindled a little further every time the door opened.

"Okay," the doctor said, "please wait outside. Don't get dressed."

I was in this tiny little hallway with two chairs shoved between supply carts, with barely enough room for anyone to pass. I had to keep turning sideways to allow people to walk by. It seemed endless. They gave me that half smile as they passed—actually, more like an "I'm so sorry" look. I waited and waited. And waited. Then they told me they wanted to do a mammogram.

A mammogram? Not a good sign. I was only thirty-three. I'd had a mammogram once before, when I was thirty, to examine a lump on the other breast. That had been benign, a fibroadenoma. I told myself this was probably the same thing. But there was that feeling in the pit of my stomach. The doctor said it was probably nothing, just another fibroadenoma.

They asked me to wait for the technician to set up the mammogram. So I waited and waited and waited until finally it was done. After what seemed like another eternity, the doctor finally called me into his office. He put a film up on one of those X-ray light boxes.

"There are some microcalcifications here in the breast," he told me.

"I don't know what a microcalcification is, but it doesn't sound good."

"I don't think it's much of anything," he said. "There's a fifty percent chance that it's fine. There's a fifty percent chance that it's precancerous cells, although typically we see those in women much older than you. It's really nothing to worry about. However, you should see a surgeon to be a hundred percent certain."

I didn't like this doctor very much.

At least I liked the surgeon. She had done the earlier biopsy, and she had given me good news. And I didn't go alone; I brought Kevin as my reinforcement. When I arrived, she looked like a happy little camper. It must be good news. She examined me and took out a really big needle and stuck it into the first lump. Fluid drew up into the syringe.

"That's a good thing!" she exclaimed. "That's a clogged milk duct, which happens sometimes after pregnancy."

Now I was feeling pretty good. Wow, maybe it really was all right! Then she stuck the needle into the second lump. No fluid. She tried again. No such luck—no fluid.

"Okay, you can get dressed."

She waited with Kevin in her office while I got dressed. When I joined them, they were having a light, seemingly uneventful conversation. Then she shoved the films into her own lighted box and, still fairly upbeat, said, "Yes, I'm pretty certain it's cancer."

BAM! SMACK! SMASH!

There really is no way to describe what it's like to hear those words. There must be some mistake. Both Dr. "hook" and the other mammogram guy had thought it was nothing. She pointed and explained why she thought what she thought.

"We'll have to wait for the results of the biopsy, but I'm pretty certain."

"So what happens if it is?" I asked.

"Based on the films, we'll have to do a mastectomy to remove the breast."

What? Wait a minute. What? What, what? Slow down. Why do we have to remove the whole breast? Just take out the lump!

"It appears as if the cancer is in three out of four quadrants. When it's in more than one quadrant, the disease is more extensive, and your best chance for survival is to have a mastectomy. Let's see what the biopsy shows, and then we can make the final decision. I would like to see you in five days."

Five more days of torture. I didn't really want to tell anyone, because I didn't want to make it real. Five days later, we met with her again.

"Yes, you have cancer," she confirmed. "I'm very sorry. I would like to schedule the surgery as quickly as possible. You will need to see a plastic surgeon specializing in breast reconstruction, as well."

Two surgeons. Lucky me. I didn't realize I was so special that I would get two surgeons. "Well, I've always thought about having some plastic surgery for maybe a nose job or some lipo, but why for this?" I asked.

"I remove the breast and the cancer. The plastic surgeon will explain your options for how you'd like your breast to look afterward. Some people actually do nothing, but you can decide after you review your options."

I imagined the boob being lopped off like an arm in a Monty Python flick. The flesh and blood would be exposed, but the doctor would say, in a heavy British accent, "That's okay. It's just a flesh wound. You've got another!"

The plastic surgeon had a new technique called a "tram-flap" mastectomy, in which muscle and tissue is taken from the patient's stomach and used to fill in the breast—sort of like a tummy tuck and a new breast at the same time. Wow, while he's in there, do you think he can tweak the nose, do some lipo, and a lube job, too?

This couldn't be real. I was only thirty-three. I had a baby, for God's sake. Oh, my God, was I going to die? Someone please wake me up from this nightmare.

Chapter Four

THE CRAZIOLOGIST

I arrived early for the appointment with the plastic surgeon, so I went across the street to look around in an antique store. Shopping makes everyone feel better, doesn't it? That was when I saw her: a beautiful bronze fountain featuring a Grecian goddess pouring from her pitcher. She was magnificent.

"What do you think?" I asked my husband.

"It's not exactly in our price range," he said, "but if it means that much to you and you really want it, we can get it."

He never could say no to me. Poor guy. He would probably buy me the Eiffel Tower if I asked him nicely. We left empty-handed and walked back in time for our appointment.

The plastic surgeon was revolting. He had no personality. He matter-of-factly went through a very thorough description of the surgery, using diagrams that were meaningless to me. Then he showed me a picture he was terribly proud of. He actually smiled. It was a picture of a breast sliced the way you would slice an orange, then sewn up with large, ugly stitches. Looking at it straight on, it reminded me of a ball with baseball stitching across it.

Excuse me. Do you have any idea what it's like to be thirty-three and told you're going to have a breast that looks like a baseball? It's one thing to hear you're going to have a mastectomy. It's quite another to *see* it. I left the office without another word.

It was a gorgeous day out. I looked up at the bright blue sky. Before that moment, I would have been smiling and taking in that beautiful view. But an indescribable, powerful dark storm swirled inside. I made it to the sidewalk and leaned with my hand against a streetlamp as I fought nausea and dizziness. Kevin stood on one side, and my mom on the other, as I retched. My two soldiers. Like two people at a funeral holding up the mother who had just lost her child.

Hey, wait a minute. People didn't throw up until they *started* chemotherapy. I looked up and saw the bronze statue in the window across the street. *Wouldn't it be nice,* I thought, *if I could just pour out the fear, pour out the cancer, the way she's pouring out her pitcher of water?* Suddenly, the statue didn't seem so important. Kevin and Mom knew there was nothing to be said. Nothing could make it seem okay. I was going to lose my breast. I was going to be sliced in half, from one side of my abdomen to the other, and restuffed like the scarecrow from *The Wizard of Oz.* And I might not even make it to Oz.

At one point, someone asked if I had spoken to an oncologist yet. Never having been through cancer with anyone, I asked, "What's an oncologist?"

What a boob I was.

"The person who handles the chemotherapy," I was told.

I felt like a moron. How could I not know that? I didn't want to believe there was a chance I might need chemotherapy, so I hadn't researched that yet. I guess the doctors didn't want me to think too far past the surgery, either, because they never mentioned it.

The one person with whom I would be connected for the next year, more so even than with my own family, was someone I hadn't even known existed. There was a whole new vocabulary and so many different kinds of doctors. I was about to become educated about all of them: breast surgeon (not to be confused with breast plastic surgeon), radiologist, hematologist, oncologist, and phlebotomist. And then there's the craziologist … oh, right. That's me.

Fortunately, I had a really good experience with the plastic surgeon I finally chose. I felt good about him when I walked into this gorgeous office on Park Avenue with spectacular, bright, "happy" artwork. When I asked who the artist was, I was told it had been painted by the surgeon. Someone as talented as this was who I wanted to do my surgery. Later I thought about the word "painting." What words are in there? *Pain-tings.* As in, there will be a lot of pain? Or the artist suffered through a lot to make the *ting.* If that wasn't a message about what to expect, I didn't know what would be.

The surgeon was kind, compassionate, and caring and took his time explaining in a very nice way how the surgery would be. He had the bedside manner the first plastic surgeon lacked. He showed me a picture of another patient. His method didn't require baseball stitching. In fact, he removed the nipple—*ouch!*—and did all the work through the hole so there wouldn't be a huge scar across the entire breast. The stomach scar would be there, but it remained below the bikini line.

I knew in an instant he was the right guy. Although I still wasn't happy about what was going to happen, I felt a whole lot better than with the first guy. At least I felt in good hands with this surgeon. The kindness alone made all the difference.

All these appointments made this into a five-week-long process before the surgery. Five weeks of torture—okay, that's fine. I decided to buy the statue. Who needs a psychologist when there's retail therapy?

The breast surgeon came highly recommended by the president of my company. She was at the top of her field, so he pulled a few strings to get me in. She would be going on vacation, so she gave me her colleague, who had a reputation as number two. I waited over seven hours to see him.

That was the first clue. You shouldn't have to wait seven hours to see the *Pope*. This same surgeon, who had such a grand reputation and in whom I had so much confidence, canceled three days before my surgery. Apparently, he had to move apartments that day, which appeared to be a bit more important than perhaps *saving my life*.

Imagine that. You have cancer and suffer all the emotional stuff, finally come to terms with it, go through all the research and decision making to pick a surgeon, put your life in his hands, prepare for surgery, and then, three days before your life is about to change, are told the surgeon has more important things to do. And because of his busy schedule, he isn't able to fit you in for weeks.

I just about lost it. I begged him to do it. Nope. Instead, I was assigned a newly graduated surgeon just off her residency.

That should have been my second clue that something might go terribly wrong.

Five weeks after the diagnosis, it was time. We arrived at the hospital at the crack of dawn, and after all the customary presurgical paperwork, I was escorted to the second stage. A new procedure, called sentinel node mapping, was being done. The goal was to remove as few lymph nodes as possible. Cancer typically makes a path from the tumor to the lymph nodes, like a path cleared by a snow plow after a storm. The storm motif is kind of appropriate here.

At the time, this mapping was about 75 percent effective in determining which lymph nodes the cancer would appear in. It also pointed out the lead, or sentinel, node—the one the cancer would most likely target. This allowed the surgeons to take out only one lymph node and do a biopsy while I was on the table.

If the sentinel lymph node was malignant, they would remove the rest of the nodes to determine how many had been affected. That in turn, would determine the prognosis. If the sentinel node was benign, they wouldn't take out any additional nodes. That scenario would lead to a better recovery and a better prognosis.

Lying on my back, I waited for my map. Kevin was by my side, holding my hand and being reassuring. I lay there in my sexy little hospital gown with my head cranked around so I could look up at a monitor. My left arm was raised over my head. Little did I know that this would be the last time I would ever be able to lift my arm above my head. Sadly, it's the little things in life that we miss in each moment.

The radiologist pointed to a spot on the monitor. How could they really tell one thing from another? Didn't it just look like some kind of messy soup?

"Here's the tumor and here are the lymph nodes," he said. I had no clue what the difference was.

"I'm going to inject this solution into the tumor," he continued. "Hopefully, by the time your surgery begins, the dye will slowly have made its way to the sentinel node and it can be biopsied."

He explained that I would feel a little pressure and then I would be taken to the pre-op area.

"Not to worry," he said. "You don't have to wait here. You won't see anything now, anyway."

He was wrong—very wrong. Within seconds, that dye flew from the tumor straight up to the lymph node. He was speechless. That wasn't good.

"I guess that means the cancer is in the nodes if it traveled that quickly," I said.

"Uh, no. Uh, it usually doesn't happen like that," he stammered.

Okay, dude, I thought, *I know it's not cool.*

I said nothing. No need to make him feel more uncomfortable. I looked at Kevin, and tears welled up in our eyes. He squeezed my hand. He knew, too.

* * *

The last thing I remember was being a little loopy, kissing Kevin and my mom, and asking them to make sure Kelsey knew how much I loved her in case I didn't come back. Then nothing. I don't even remember drifting off to sleep. It was as if one second I was awake and the next, nothing.

Then I was in a dream. I could barely open my eyes. Some kind of light broke through. I didn't know where I was or what was happening. Had I died? Were those the lights you saw when you died? I couldn't figure out what was going on. Then I was in a panic, the lights were going faster and faster, and I was sliding through a tunnel.

Had I died? You're supposed to feel light and airy and beautiful when you die. Aren't you? You see the light and go to it. Isn't that the way it works? I didn't feel light and airy. I felt terrified. Why was I having so much trouble trying to speak? I kept asking, *What's happening?* I heard voices and knew they were right beside me, but they weren't responding. I couldn't see them.

What's happening? Still nothing. Where was I? *Please help me.* I was so cold. Something was terribly wrong. *Please tell me what's happening!* Was I dead? Were they taking me to the morgue because they didn't know I was still alive? They kept on with their ridiculous chatter. They were complaining about something, but who were they and where was I? *God, help me, please.* They ignored me. I was so cold, my body was shaking.

It got worse. I was convulsing. *Please, I'm so cold, please help me, I feel so sick. I'm going to throw up, but I can't move.* My body was convulsing, yet I couldn't control it. My eyes could open barely a sliver, and only for a second before they closed again. All I could see were lights through a haze. *What happened? Was I in an accident?* Every bump, every movement, was a horrible trauma to my body—a body that was not my own.

Am I paralyzed? Why can't I remember anything? What's happening? My body felt like lead. The agony, the weight of it, was like having bricks piled on top of me, like during the witch hunts of old. I was being pressed to death.

"Where am I?" My mouth moved.

Finally, a response—the first and last. A voice from the fog. "You're going to recovery," she snapped.

Recovery? The word didn't register.

"Please, I'm so cold. Please help me."

Nothing. No response. The trip took hours. Recovery? What was I recovering from?

Recovery. It all came back. I had wandered in a fog at first, then was hit with an enormous wave. Like an innocent child who joyfully wades into the ocean only to be flipped and tumbled mercilessly without being able to catch her breath. It washed over me, flooded through me in an instant: the panic, the fear, the reality. The horrible reality. Cancer.

I was no longer in a dream. I was tumbling in the wave. I couldn't breathe, couldn't come up for air. Those three words pounded in my head: *You have cancer. I have cancer. Please just let me go back to sleep. Maybe if I do, and I wake up again, it won't be real. I won't have cancer and it will all have been a dream.*

There was never a moment in my life when I felt more terrified and alone. Two heartless people who obviously had never gone through anything like this were in control of the most traumatic moment of my life. How could they be so cruel? They really didn't care. They were ignoring me. *Hello! I really am alive!* We crashed through another door … more trauma, more pain. *Oh, God, please don't let them bang into anything.* Bang!

The movement. I was horribly sick. The bright lights, the noise, so much going on. I couldn't process it all. I barely opened my eyes before they closed again against my will. I whimpered because I couldn't cry. That would have been too much for my body to handle. *Please, God, help me. Where's Kevin? Where's my mom? I need them. They'll help. Oh, Kelsey. Please, God. Please let this stop.*

The mean one spoke with an attitude. "Where do you want her?"

At last, there was hope; someone else was here. Maybe they would help me. My teeth hurt from chattering; my jaw ached; my head was pounding from the gnashing of my teeth. Everything, all my senses, seemed in a heightened state.

"Please, I'm so cold. What's happening?" I whispered.

A kinder voice spoke. Tubes were everywhere. I couldn't move my body voluntarily, and yet I was convulsing.

"Please don't move me."

The words were barely audible even to me. I thought I was dying. I didn't think I was going to make it. I couldn't imagine anything worse happening to my body and being able to handle it.

Then it got worse, much worse. The nausea grew and grew. *Oh, God, please keep it down or let me throw up—anything to make it better.*

"Please, where is my family?"

"We can't let them in yet," the kind voice responded.

Oh, God, maybe you should just take me now. I can't bear it any longer.

Kelsey. I loved her so much, but I didn't think I could do this, even for her. How would she live without me? The thought was too much. I *could* do it for her. *No. Oh, God, I don't think I can. Please make it stop.*

I could only stay on the same thought for a few seconds. Everything rushed around in my head, spinning, looping. Split seconds of thoughts, tumbling over each other. Wild, crazy, all-over-the-place thoughts. Please, God, help me. I just wanted to curl into a fetal position and cry, but my body wouldn't move. Had something gone wrong? Was I paralyzed? There wasn't a part of me that I could move. My heart felt as if it were jumping out of my chest, but my body felt dead.

I was exhausted, but I was in and out, and my voice was barely audible. I was crying, whimpering, but mostly inside, because I couldn't really cry. It was too painful. No one ever told me any of this would happen.

"Please, my family—where are they?" I whispered.

"They can't come in for a while, dear."

I was losing blood. They needed to do a transfusion. What happened to me? Someone was lying on top of me. They were placing bricks on me as they had in the witch hunt days. What was that from? I had read a book about that, or was it in a movie? I think I read it in school, in *The Crucible*. They placed a board on top of the witch and, one by one, added stones. That's what was happening to me.

Was it in the lymph nodes? I needed to know. That question kept hitting me again and again, making my head spin. Was it in the lymph nodes? How much longer before my family could come in? How long before I could have my answers?

They kept doing things to me. Tubes, pumps, machines. Oh, the sounds…

"She needs more blood."

Oh, no, what's happening now? I didn't have enough blood. Would my family be able to donate? I didn't think so; there was some kind of problem. *Please let me fall asleep.* Maybe I wouldn't feel the pain, wouldn't feel the bricks. But that was impossible. How can it be that you hear but can't respond? My mind was fuzzy, very fuzzy, in and out. I felt as if my brain were disconnected from my voice and my body, yet still connected to the pain and numbness and nausea.

The surgery had been scheduled to take six hours, but complications had arisen. It had taken ten and a half hours. Of course, I didn't remember. The last thing I remembered was being a little loopy.

Chapter Five

HIT BY A TRUCK—NO, MAKE THAT *THREE* TRUCKS

Meanwhile, back in the waiting room, the support troops had gathered. About twenty people had come throughout the day, and many more had been calling. Kathy said they had needed rolls and rolls of quarters because they weren't allowed to use cell phones in the hospital. How awesome to know that so many people cared! They had trekked all the way into the city to be there for me and my family. The social worker talked to them regularly to give them encouragement, and then the surgeon finally came out and let them know what had happened.

Hours later, I heard familiar voices. It was Kevin and my mom. There's no describing that moment. I felt like a child: I needed her comfort, her reassurance, to make it all go away. I had the urge to call her "Mommy." Mommies always make it better.

I felt their concern, though. They were trying to remain upbeat.

"Something's wrong," I said. "I'm so cold. Please help me."

I felt so sick. I needed them to help me, to make it better. But they couldn't help. All they could do was explain what was going on. My eyes would open for a split second, but I didn't really see anything. It was as though the weight of my eyelids was just too much to lift.

Kevin's voice told me everything. "The surgery took much longer than expected, honey. There were some complications, but everything is going to be okay. You've been losing blood and they're giving you more. You have to stay in recovery until they have the blood loss and the nausea under control."

Mom was painfully quiet.

"Please, can you help me?" I said. "I can't take it anymore."

Kevin walked away for a while, then returned. "I'm sorry," he said. "They can't give you anything more. You'll have to wait because they've already given you all they're allowed."

I whimpered, "Was it in my lymph nodes?"

Kevin paused. He didn't want to say, but I already knew the answer. He choked up and tried to keep his voice from cracking. "Yes. I'm so sorry, honey." He kissed my head and squeezed my hand. "It's in the lymph nodes."

Nothing else mattered. Everything went black. My mind just couldn't handle any other thoughts. It was in the lymph nodes. I wanted to cry, but that would have been too much for my body to endure. It was in the lymph nodes. It was much worse than we'd hoped. It was in the lymph nodes—that changed everything.

At three o'clock in the morning, I was rolled to my room. I had been at the hospital since six o'clock yesterday morning. The room was dark. We passed someone in the other bed. There was still no relief. I had thought that going to the room, where it was quieter, would help, but the trip from recovery only seemed to make it worse. How would I make it through the night?

Sadly, one thing the hospital had was plenty of clocks. One hung on the wall directly in front of my eyes, so when I was able to open them even a little, that was what I saw. I could always measure exactly how little time had passed since I last opened my eyes.

※　＊　＊

I thought I was going to die right here and now. *Please, God, Mary, just get me through the next minute, the next few seconds.* I couldn't even say a

Hail Mary or an Our Father. My mind couldn't focus enough. I just kept repeating, *Mary, please get me through the next minute. It's in the lymph nodes. Hail Mary, full of grace … Hail Mary, full of grace … Hail Mary, full of grace. It's in the lymph nodes.*

I thought I might die. I actually felt as if I could bear no more and was losing the will to stay alive. My body couldn't endure anything more, and the thoughts kept going through my head: *I am probably going to die anyway. Why try so hard to stay alive now? I should just let go. At least the pain will stop.*

That was one of those horrible moments when even the thought of my beautiful child wasn't enough to overcome the trauma. Even she couldn't give me the will to live. When Princess Diana was in the accident, everyone had expected her last words to be, "Please tell my boys I love them." Instead, she had said, "I can't breathe." That's how I felt.

Mary, I thought, *I don't want to die, but I might if you don't carry me through the next minute.* I still felt the crushing weight, the numbness, the nausea, and the pain bearing down, getting worse minute by minute. The medication wasn't working. Wasn't it supposed to make the pain go away? The nurse arrived.

"Please, more pain medication," I whispered. It was a huge exertion to get the words out.

"No," the nurse said. "The massive pain medication you were given during the surgery is wearing off. What we have isn't as strong. There's nothing I can give you that's strong enough to help."

I was moaning, and I kept from crying because that made it so much worse. I felt as though I were dying. *I'm going to die all alone in this horrible darkness, in a hospital, without my family,* I thought. So I kept asking Mary for her help. The clock ticked through the night. I was sleepless, filled only with the slow and agonizing torture. It was as close to death as I could imagine being, as close to hell as I ever wanted to be. For the first time in my life, I really thought I could die. And for the first time in my life, I could have let it happen.

✻ ✻ ✻

Daybreak didn't improve things, but at least there was sunlight. I could feel the rays in the room. It seemed like a beautiful summer day—a sharp contrast to the darkness I felt inside. A parade of people came in and out, but I didn't open my eyes; it was just too much effort. My family took turns coming up to see me. There was comfort in that, even if they only sat quietly next to the bed.

Well, having a party was more like it. Fortunately, there were always jokes and stories. At one point, ten of them had crammed into the room. I opened my eyes for a second and felt comfort knowing they were there, but it was too hard to communicate. I just didn't have the strength.

The doctor arrived and explained what had transpired. The surgery had been much more extensive than expected. My body had undergone much more trauma than anticipated. They'd had to remove more than they hoped, because the sentinel node biopsy showed cancer in the lymph nodes.

They hadn't expected that there wouldn't be enough tummy tissue for the reconstruction. A partial implant had been inserted to make up the difference. Tubes and drains filled with blood and mucus came out of my abdomen, chest, and side. My mother told the doctor that I probably feel as if I'd been hit by a truck. The doctor said, quite seriously and sympathetically, "Actually, it feels more like she got hit by *three* trucks."

That summed up how I felt. Later I found out that I'd had a very bad reaction to the anesthesia, which caused the convulsions and nausea. The defining thing, though, was the excruciating pain—and the realization that my body was no longer the one I'd spent the past thirty-three years in.

My body was no longer my own. Several days passed before I was able to get out of bed. Although this surgery was normally quite painful, mine was exceptionally so. In an effort to get whatever abdominal tissue they could to fill the breast, they had pulled my stomach so tight I couldn't stand up straight.

It was so awful. My family sneaked my baby up just to bring me some joy. She looked *so* cute—that adorable little cherub face with the huge chipmunk cheeks. She had one arm and one leg hanging over the side of the stroller as she watched me try to get out of bed for the first time.

I grunted and groaned while people moved my legs over the edge of the mattress. They lifted me by my hands, which was excruciating since it pulled on my arm and the whole surgical site. Then they set my feet on the floor, with me bent in half the whole time. She looked at me and started chuckling at how funny I must have looked. She appeared much wiser than her eight months. Everyone laughed, and I half-smiled for the first time in days. I couldn't laugh, though—that was too painful. But I thanked God for her.

Each day, I walked, little by little, down the hospital corridor, hunched over and in excruciating pain. I resembled a centenarian with bad osteoporosis! One older man, an aide, yelled at me to stand up straight. Can you imagine the nerve? What a moron. What really came to mind was to tell him to f— off. Cursing wasn't very ladylike, but there are times when nothing else has quite the same impact.

Eight days later, I was finally able to go home. The hour-and-a-half trip on New York's worst highways set me back again. Once home, I realized that walking up the stairs to the second-floor bedroom was impossible. No one realizes how crucial stomach muscles are until abdominal surgery comes along. I was unable to sleep in a bed, because it wouldn't raise my body and legs the way a hospital bed does. So the family room on the main floor became my bedroom. The sofa lounge was moved in there; it was the most comfortable thing we had. I slept in that for nearly four months, until I could lie on my side in a bed again.

* * *

The painkillers were a joke. I ran out of medication on a Friday. Kevin talked with the doctor on call. "No, sorry, she can't have any more," he said.

"She's in excruciating pain," my husband pleaded. "You have to give her something."

"No, sorry, she can't have any more. If you want, you can call the doctor on Monday. If they say it's okay, you can have more."

That was not a good answer. Clearly, when they prescribed it they hadn't considered how much worse than usual the surgery had been, and they hadn't factored in my low pain threshold. An assistant had done the discharge, and I guess my doctor didn't review the paperwork. I had to use Lamaze breathing techniques to get through the pain, minute by minute.

Kevin lit candles so I could focus on them while I tried to meditate. I don't know why I thought that would work. I'd never been able to focus that way before—what made me think I could meditate while in agony? The pain consumed me. Getting through every moment became my entire existence that weekend.

On Sunday, my brother, Richie, called. "Get that doctor on the phone," he said, "and tell him you need pain medication, and you take as much as you need to make it better."

That seemed like sound advice. We were still so naive about some things. I didn't want to overdose, but obviously I had an extremely low pain threshold. So Kevin called again and told them they had to page the doctor.

The doctor called us directly. "Of course you can have it," he said. "You shouldn't have to live with that pain."

Another lesson: don't take no for an answer when you know in your heart that you need something.

My progress was slow—much slower than I'd expected. I measured my progress by how many times I was able to walk around the pool in our yard. The first try after being home for a week, I couldn't even make it once.

My dad was very encouraging. He would call or stop by every day to see how many laps around the pool I'd done. Thank goodness it was summertime! I couldn't bear to have anything touch or sit against my stomach, so my mother and Diane bought me several huge, smock-type dresses, the same kind my grandmother had worn.

The absolutely worst part was that my beautiful eight-month-old child couldn't come near me. Babies are very active at that age. They love to kick their feet and flap their arms, which makes them all the cuter—but I couldn't risk her kicking or hitting me. I wanted to scoop her up and make her laugh, but the slightest touch to my upper torso was agony. Just for me to get a kiss, someone had to hold her arms and lean her over me.

When colder weather arrived, I wore stretchy maternity pants and loose-fitting shirts. I felt so much older than my thirty-three years—like an invalid, in fact. My body was not my own. No one had warned me it would be like this.

*   *   *

Only one thing was worse than being diagnosed with cancer: being told I couldn't have any more children.

About two weeks after the surgery, I had my first appointment with the oncologist. I chose the oncologist with the most experience treating younger women still in their child-bearing years. I liked her a lot, but I did usually wait a good four to five hours for each appointment—not great when I felt the way I did and had traveled nearly two hours to get there.

During the appointments, we reviewed my treatment plan and discussed whatever approach would allow me to have a child after the treatments were over. Six kids was my magic number. Kevin wanted four kids, so we'd settled on five. I was already thirty-three, so I wanted to get started as soon as possible after I healed, which I expected would take about six months (Yes, I was optimistic.)

I couldn't wait to hear the pitter-patter of little feet and feel the fullness of having children all around me in our home. Six months would go by quickly. My big question for the doctor was, "How long after the treatments can I start trying to have a child?"

The response was not what I expected.

"It's not really recommended after this diagnosis," she said. "Particularly since this was in your lymph nodes and was diagnosed shortly after you gave birth. We consider your cancer to be pregnancy related. You take a great risk getting pregnant again. Our hope is to keep you from going into menopause. If you're healthy five years down the road, then we'll look at your options again. But I don't think you should consider getting pregnant—ever. It's just too risky."

BOOM! That couldn't possibly be right. I didn't just hear that. No, it couldn't be right. Then I looked at Kevin. He clasped his hands in his lap and focused on them. I saw the tears in his eyes and knew he felt it, too. Having more children had been my reason to heal as quickly as possible. It had been my reason for *everything*.

There had to be a way. "What about saving my eggs?" I asked.

"I'm afraid that isn't possible, either," the doctor said. "In order to harvest your eggs, you'd have hormone injections to boost your egg production. Since this cancer is pregnancy related, the injections would also create risk that the cancer would grow."

That was it—all my hopes and dreams shattered in one conversation.

When I had been diagnosed, I looked at it as a business transaction. I had always been very goal oriented, so I set getting better as my goal. I would have the treatments and move on. My chances for recurrence were only 15 to 20 percent. Those were pretty good odds. Doubt gnawed at me, and I did have some fear, but that was natural. But this … this was much more definitive.

"It's just too risky." The doctor looked at my husband and my mother. "I really don't think she should do this. Please try to convince her."

This diagnosis was infinitely worse than the cancer. Having children was what I had looked forward to my whole adult life. The cancer was temporary; I didn't really expect it to have a lasting impact other than the scars. But this diagnosis was permanent. My whole future had been altered in one sentence.

*   *   *

I left the oncologist's office not caring about anything else she had said. I didn't care what would happen during the treatments. I was fresh out of optimism. For three weeks, I cried, anywhere and everywhere. Just when I thought I had sobbed myself dry, I cried some more. Physically, I was incapacitated. Emotionally, I was dead.

It hurt to cry, but I didn't care. Maybe the physical pain would distract me from the pain in my heart. There was no consoling me. Nothing anyone could say would make this better. I always tried to see what good might come of a bad situation, but there was nothing here. I had nothing left.

Then, when I was completely drained from all the crying and the surgery and dealing with the new physical me and the scars and limitations, and when I didn't care about anything anymore because my dreams had been shattered, salt was thrown on the wounds: it was time to start chemotherapy.

It was a little frightening at first—the unknown of how I would really fare—but at least I wouldn't die … . Well, I *thought* I wouldn't.

Many people have gone through chemotherapy and fared well. I thought I was a fairly strong person. Other people even told me that. I could work a hundred hours a week, I had been a competitive swimmer, and I was the mother of an infant—I had even delivered her naturally. So I must be strong, right?

Well, chemo did me in. It was no cakewalk. Yes, I'd been warned I would lose my hair and feel nauseated, but there really was no preparing for the real thing. When you have a stomach virus, it lasts a day, maybe two, and God knows, you don't believe you'll get through it. You temporarily lose the knowledge of what it's like not to feel sick. But the sickness that came with chemo was like food poisoning that lasted for months.

Dad had gone back to Florida. Kevin and Mom stuck around, as usual—my army, my strength, my comfort. So after I waited the customary five hours for the appointment, the doctor explained that a very aggressive treatment was recommended given my youth and the fact that I had a form of cancer that was especially aggressive in several ways. Moreover, the younger you are, the worse the prognosis.

I didn't quite need to hear that one. I thought it would be the opposite: the younger you are, the stronger you are. But that's not what the statistics show. The doctor also believed this would be the best course to keep me from going into premature menopause.

I would have ACT chemotherapy, short for Adriamycin, Cytoxan, and Taxol. I would have it every two weeks instead of three. The quicker the treatments, the theory went, the less time the reproductive organs had to get damaged. Adriamycin, by the way, is endearingly known as the "red death."

Chapter Six

THE OLD MAN
IS SNORING: CHEMO

The nurses were all very nice and explained I would feel something going into my vein and then probably taste it in my throat. They weren't going to leave, because I might go into anaphylactic shock and they needed to be ready to give me an injection. Okay, so maybe I *would* die after all.

I thought I was doing all right because I didn't go into anaphylactic shock as soon as they began pumping me full of chemicals. I got a little confident. Maybe this wouldn't be so bad after all. But all the explanations in the world couldn't prepare me for what was to come.

The nausea began while I was still hooked up to the IV bags. It was mild at first, but it kept getting worse as the infusion continued. I really noticed it when we went out to eat after the treatment. Normally, I really looked forward to a nice meal in one of New York City's many wonderful restaurants. When nothing appealed to me and I pushed the food away, I thought, *Well, isn't this great?* It wasn't supposed to set in *this* quickly.

And that was the best I was going to feel for several months. We made it home, and I slept and slept and slept. Mom had to go back to Florida for a week to straighten some things out. She had expected to stay in New York for only a couple of weeks, to help with the birth of my goddaughter; then I was diagnosed. It had been almost three months since she arrived. She was a superwoman.

The fatigue set in. By the fifth day, I went to the store with my friend Diane, just to get out. I had to get past the idea that I looked like an L-bracket used to hang shelves, because I still couldn't stand up straight. I wanted to look for something other than the three granny-style housedresses I'd been in for a month.

Who would have thought a walk from the car to the store's entrance would be so draining? I felt as if my body were loaded with lead. Then my head started to hurt. We never even made it to the front door of the store. No new dress for me. I went home and straight to the family room, but I couldn't get comfortable. In fact, it was worse than usual, if that was even possible.

Something was awfully wrong, but I didn't know what. My head was pounding, and the pain medication did nothing to relieve it. I just whimpered because crying hurt my head too much.

Around eleven that evening, Kevin kissed my forehead. "You're burning up!" he said.

He took my temperature: 102. Since my normal temperature was 96.8—nearly two degrees below most people's—the fever was more like 104. Not good when you're undergoing chemo.

"Do you remember what they said about that?" Kevin asked. "If you have a fever over a hundred, we have to call."

They said to get to the hospital immediately. Kelsey was asleep already, as expected for any eleven-month-old. So there I went again, calling friends for another emergency, this time in the middle of the night. Diane had been asleep but made it to my house in five minutes. She showed up in her nightgown and sneakers. What a friend!

"Don't worry, don't worry," she said, "I'll take care of everything."

"What about getting up with your kids?" I asked weakly.

"My mom will come first thing in the morning so Curt can leave for work."

I felt guilty imposing on her entire family like this, but I felt too awful, I had to let it go.

The hour-and-a-half car ride was more torture. As it was, I couldn't sit comfortably in a car since the surgery. Added to that was the pounding in my head, and the ache in every atom of my body.

We had no idea where to go, because it was our first visit to that hospital for anything except surgery. We found our way down to the basement, and I had to lie down. I couldn't even walk or stand or sit in the wheelchair.

Within minutes, the emergency room doctor said I had a neutropenic fever. I would be admitted immediately and put on IV antibiotics. My white blood count was below 200. A normal white blood count was between 4,300 and 10,800. If I caught any type of infection, my body wouldn't be able to fight it. I would die.

"How many treatments have you had?" the doctor asked.

"Just one," I said.

"Wow," he said. "This doesn't usually happen this quickly."

What a surprise: *moi,* a little more sensitive than most. I didn't want to talk, and I didn't care what *he* wanted to do—I just needed someone to make me feel better.

"Please give me something for the headache," I said.

"We can't give you anything that might bring the fever down. We can only treat you with antibiotics and IV fluids."

So that was it? I was just supposed to deal with it? This was no ordinary headache. There are no words to describe the extent of it. I had suffered before with horrible daily headaches and migraines to boot. This wasn't even in the same league. It was the kind of pain where you can't open your eyes, you can't talk or move your head, and you just want to cry but even that hurts too much. It clamped down like a huge vise on my entire head and neck. My head felt as though it weighed a thousand pounds.

It was worse than a migraine because along with this headache, the rest of my body hurt, too. All I wanted was for someone to cut my head off and throw it away. I would have paid a million dollars and given my next child for an Advil. (My firstborn was a keeper, and they wouldn't know I couldn't have a second, so it was a safe trade.) The noise was deafening and intensified the pain. I needed earplugs to block out some of that painful racket. They didn't have any.

It was well after daybreak before I finally got a room. I kept begging for an Advil or Tylenol or anything for the pain. "Not yet. I'm sorry," they chanted.

My sister, Kathy, my sister-in-law, Barbara, and friends Diane and Cathy came. I couldn't talk to them. I couldn't even open my eyes. It was too painful, so I lay there in agony as they talked. I loved them all dearly and was grateful for them being there for support, but I couldn't bear to have people talking nearby, and I didn't know how to tell them.

The only thing I could ask was that my sister not call our mom—I didn't want her flying right back up again. She promised she wouldn't. I stayed in the hospital a few more days until my white blood count came back up, although it remained dangerously low. They kept me on antibiotics and said I needed to discuss the future treatments with my oncologist. The admitting doctor wasn't even sure I'd be able to *have* any more treatments. At last, they sent me home.

* * *

After a four-hour wait, we were ushered into the oncologist's office. Rather than stop the treatments, she would cut the chemo back to 25 percent. If everything went well, they would increase the amounts as we went along until, hopefully, we made it back to the full level.

The next issue was my white blood count, which never really recovered from the neutropenic fever. So I would give myself Neupogen shots to build up the count. The unfortunate side effect to that treatment is bone pain.

It's easy to say, "The side effect is bone pain." It's quite another to actually feel it. There was no relief for this agony. It felt as though the bones were crunching against each another. The ache went right down to the marrow. There were times I couldn't even get off the sofa, yet it was too painful to simply lie there. We tried baths and painkillers, but it was another thing I just had to deal with. And since the treatments were cumulative, so were the pain and nausea. You got it! They just kept getting worse and worse. The pain and nausea consumed me, and I did my best to try meditating to help alleviate them. Even though I wasn't feeling the least bit motivated, I also felt I *needed* to make some type of effort toward healing the cancer. One of the things that helped was when my friend Joanne sent me a few of Dr. Bernie Siegel's tapes. There was no way to quiet my mind, and I could handle only a couple of minutes at a time, so the visualization recordings were a much easier way to help me feel that I was doing something toward healing.

At the biweekly blood tests, I held my breath. Would they be able to continue the treatments? If I didn't have the treatments, what would my chances drop to? My white blood count remained in the dangerously low range. I was extremely weak and growing weaker. The fatigue grew worse. I was able to do less and less. Getting dressed was a challenge, and I was sleeping seventeen hours a day.

Then the cough set in—persistent, draining, and worrisome, since it could mean the cancer had spread to my lungs. The cough was relentless and exhausting. Then the concern was pneumonia. "It has been a terrible assault on your body," the doctor said of the surgery and the treatments, especially since there was no recovery time between treatments.

The effects made me cranky, and I couldn't think straight. I felt cluttered and couldn't perform the simplest tasks. It was all too much, and I didn't know where to start. The nausea radiated up from the pit of my stomach to my chest, the back of my throat, and into my mouth and nose. A metallic taste stayed in my mouth, and I couldn't get rid of it, no matter what I put on my tongue or how many times I brushed my teeth.

The awful taste continued along with what felt like little throbbing bursts from my neck, through my ears and skull, pulsating, *thump, thump, thump.* I couldn't stand the smell of anything, but I wanted to eat something to make it feel better, to make it stop, but nothing did. My body did not want to move, my head felt full of fuzz, and I had cottonmouth. I'd had cottonmouth from imbibing the occasional one too many, but this time someone stuffed my entire head with cotton and threw in a nice, fuzzy fog for kicks.

It felt like a weight in my head, as if the top third of my skull were full of concrete and ready to burst. It was almost impossible to describe—I could actually *feel* the chemicals in my brain. I had a rush of diarrhea. But no, it wouldn't come out. Now constipation. Even my poop couldn't make up its mind!

I just wanted to go to bed, but my heart was racing and I couldn't sleep. So what to do? Sleep or run around the block? Oh, no, that's right—I couldn't even walk up the stairs. Feeling this horrible, I certainly wasn't going to run around the block. With the drugs wreaking holy havoc on my body, it was the most restless sleep imaginable.

Food was definitely an issue. No one could cook food in the house. The smell of *anything* being cooked—even just warmed in the microwave or toaster oven—put me over the edge. We knew it was bad when my mother warmed a croissant and—from upstairs! —I told them a skunk had sneaked into the house. The smell was so awful, I wanted to vomit.

We don't live in the country, just the suburbs, and to this day I have never seen a skunk on Long Island, but I was certain one was in the house. That was the end of cooking anything in the house. So the poor toaster oven joined the microwave in the garage. The oven was banned as well, though it couldn't be moved without ripping up the kitchen. I have to say, though, I did give it some thought.

If anyone wanted to cook, it had to happen on the day I went into the city for my treatment, and the house had to be aired out before I got home. Ridiculous, right? But that was reality: I couldn't stomach any smells whatever, since even the faintest whiff of anything was magnified ten times, with a dump truck load of manure added for good measure. There was very little I could stomach.

A couple of months after chemo ended, the toaster oven moved back in, like the twenty-year-old child you can't seem to get rid of. I think the microwave might have been the worst casualty, the black sheep banished permanently, to be sought out only by visiting guests or for the occasional bag of popcorn on movie night. Even favorite smells like flowers were too much to handle. How sad is that?

Chapter Seven

HAIR, HAIR ... ANYWHERE?

I cut my hair really short, dyed it, and put orange/blond streaks in it. Why? I had no freakin' clue. Maybe it was *Hey, what the hell—it's going to fall out anyway, so why not go for it?* By the end of the second week after the second treatment, we celebrated Kelsey's first birthday. My close friends and family came. It must have been a real shocker to see the new style that did its best to hide the missing patches

Yup, a thirty-three-year-old woman doing the comb-over. I actually envied Donald Trump. I dare not wash it because that made it fall out faster, so I went two weeks without a shampoo. Gross. I was desperate. Bald was not a fun alternative. Let's see: greasy or bald? I'll take grease. Brushing it was also taboo, so I just kind of pushed it into place. Not washing it kept it stiff enough so that it stayed, like meringue.

My beautiful little angel was quite cute. As a mother, how do you not hug your child? At the age when she needed nurturing the most, the pain of not being able to hold her and rock her, being able only to watch her from a distance, was further anguish.

I could hold her hand and walk a little with her, but if she pulled on my arm (which one-year-olds do), the pain was tough to bear. Even with my good arm, the pulling sent pain shooting from one side over to the other. The only real way we could play was for me to get down on my hands and knees at a distance. Kelsey had started walking by now, so she lunged happily at me and grabbed my hair.

Kids always do that, but the hair doesn't usually come out. This time she got two really good fistfuls. As she looked from the clumps to me, completely bewildered, she seemed to think, *Oh, that's interesting.* Then she squealed, delighted that she had pulled my hair out. I burst out laughing—the look of utter shock followed by clarity was just too funny!

There was no question that my hair would soon be gone, so I called Diane. She always knew the right thing to say and do. She was the talented decorator; the hair, makeup, and clothing advisor; and the all-around knows-exactly-what-you-want-when-you-want-it friend who never charged a dime.

This time, I needed help picking out a wig. *Wow,* I thought, *at least this is going to be fun—I get to pick new hair!* We traveled from salon to salon, from New York City to the ends of Long Island, in search of the perfect wig. There were so many options, and none of them the least bit appealing.

I had always wanted to be a blonde. I thought, *cool, I get to be a blond. I'll look great. It'll make all the difference in the world. They do have more fun, you know.*

Big mistake. Ugh! Atrocious. Absolutely all wrong. I had never imagined that changing my hair color would be so difficult. Wrong, wrong, wrong! Next.

Then came the styles. We tried them all: short, long, flat, curly. From Dolly Parton to Dorothy Hamil to punk rocker. About the only thing I didn't try was blue. I tried anything that didn't look like me, because that was the one person I didn't want to be just now. Nothing worked. The fun was over, so I thought it would be less fun but a lot easier just to look like little old me.

Wrong again! I realized that all I really wanted was to look like myself. I didn't want to be the sick Joyce, the one with cancer. I wanted to go back to being regular Joyce—the me I'd been before all this happened. Sitting through the wig process and looking at myself again and again and again as someone else had been far from fun.

Not only was I already nauseated and extremely uncomfortable, I looked god-awful. My skin had become gray, and no amount of makeup could cover the dark circles under my eyes. I was also bald. Not the sorta sexy, 1990s Sinead O'Connor bald, but *ugly* bald. I was trapped in someone else's body. Who was this person staring back at me? I looked like the walking dead.

Diane could do wonders with makeup, but there wasn't much she could do to touch this one up. I cried. After about the fifth trip, we finally settled on two wigs, one worse than the other, and neither looking anything like me. One was short, red, and straight, and the other was a genuine disaster.

We went to a place that used natural hair that people had sold or donated. They actually made the wig for the individual customer.

The more we tried, the worse it looked. It didn't have enough curl to it, so they added more, like giving it a perm. All that did was create a scary witch hairdo, a finger-in-the-light-socket look, for the bargain-basement price of twelve hundred dollars. And even after all the work that went into making and choosing those wigs, the multiple trips, and the combined cost of over sixteen hundred dollars, I couldn't keep them on my head. They itched; they irritated; they hurt; they never fit right. They were horrible. Not to mention, they really looked pretty dreadful. Most of the time, I just did without.

I couldn't go out without anything on my head, though, because I was always so cold, especially with summer over. So I wore hats. One glorious day, I discovered a little beanie-type cap that fit snugly and could be worn under a hat. I called it my "chemo cap."

Now, one of the side effects of the chemo was that I was always freezing. Not just cold, but shaking-with-chills freezing. I had to be bundled up all the time, especially when I slept. I was exhausted, but although I dozed, I still couldn't sleep soundly. On top of the surgery and the nausea and the bone pain, I always felt weird, uncomfortable, and I could not get warm.

One day, the family was joking with my brother-in-law about his baldness, which had appeared at the ripe old age of twenty. Someone asked if it was true that bald men were colder because so much heat is lost through the head. Bingo! If their heads were bald and they were cold, and I was bald and cold, maybe my head was cold, too.

I started wearing the chemo cap at night. It was a little tough to get used to having something tight on my head while I slept, so I stretched it out. Sometimes it fell off, but let me tell you, that was the greatest gift I'd received in a while. The cause of my extreme weird feeling while sleeping had been solved. Life was good.

Okay. That lasted about thirty seconds. Menopause kicked in, and with it, the insane random hot flashes, followed shortly by hallucinations. Yup, that's right, no joke. I said hot flashes *and* hallucinations. Full-blown, chemo-induced menopause. The hallucinations? Well, that's a story all its own.

✳   ✳   ✳

It was daytime. I was still sleeping in my sofa lounge, which had been moved up to the bedroom. Hearing a noise, I opened my eyes and slowly sat up. A strange man was in my room. He was wearing all black, along with a black mask like a ninja's, and he was coming for me.

"Who are you?" I asked. "What are you doing here?"

He said nothing.

"What do you want?"

He just kept coming. I started to scream. The door opened, and Kevin rushed in to hug me.

"Get him!" I yelled.

"Who?"

"Him!"

I pointed. He was gone. Oh, my goodness. I realized that no one had been there.

Kevin hugged me. "It's okay," he said.

"No, it's not freaking okay. There was a man in my room. What's happening to me?"

Several days later, it happened again. And again and again. Different scenarios, all very real. Same result. I absolutely believed I was losing my mind. Do you suppose someone could have mentioned to me that hallucinations could be a side effect of the drugs? Ya think?

So I got my wigs. Yippee! I could look seminormal for my little girl. I got down on the floor again to play. She was absolutely fascinated by the change. *Who the heck is this woman now?* she must have wondered. *How did her hair grow back so fast?* So she lunged at me again, laughing, hands wide open. I braced myself. Yup, she pulled the whole wig off!

Bewildered, she looked in alarm at the bald-headed person, then at the wig in her chubby little hands. She shrieked with delight. This was fun! Laughing, she grabbed the whole kit and caboodle and ran—well, waddled—away as fast as she could. She had hit the jackpot, and the prize was just too good to give up.

So, you must surely be asking, what's the next crisis? Glad you asked. Remember how my white blood cell count never really recovered? Well, because of that, I never completed the full treatment plan. Which brought up the next crisis: they were concerned that I had developed leukemia. Nope, not kidding.

We began the process of ruling out leukemia and other types of cancer. That was no laughing matter. (Well, now it sort of is, because you just can't make this stuff up.) So, how to tell if I had leukemia? That's right: a bone marrow biopsy. As if all the other side effects weren't enough and I weren't in enough pain and didn't feel miserable enough, now they wanted to crunch through the bones in my lower back with a needle the size of a turkey baster. Not fun.

Then I waited—again. Five days. Thank God the diagnosis came back benign. But what was causing this problem with my white blood cells? I went to doctors and specialists at the City's and Long Island's top hospitals. Chemo was over, yet I still couldn't risk infection. My white count hovered around 1,000. I didn't want to end up back in the hospital with neutropenic fever.

It's okay, they said. Just be cautious, and don't do anything crazy like sit in a room full of people or be near anyone who's sick. *Uh, that's pretty funny—I am in a hospital, after all.*

No one had the faintest clue what was going on. Nope, they said, hadn't seen it before—until finally I had an appointment with another specialist. She ran a slew of tests that went out to the Midwest, so the results would take a few weeks. She found out I had an immune antibody, probably from the chemotherapy. You *really* can't make this stuff up.

Now, millions of people have had chemo, and I was certainly no poster child for handling it well. Many have handled it much better than I did, and new drugs help ease many of the symptoms. I imagine that others have handled it worse, too. But ultimately, I discovered why it was so much worse for me.

First, I always had been extremely sensitive. I was sick a lot as a child and got horrific hangovers even without drinking too much. Second, my body was already so toxic that any little extra thing I put into or through it added more to an already overflowing mug.

Support groups? An amazing solace for some people, but I always felt worse when I left. They really brought me down. So I trusted my instincts and realized they weren't good for me just then.

Ever had an itch you can't scratch? The thing was, mine *literally* couldn't be scratched. Every time I had an itch, I wanted to rip my skin off. I couldn't do anything, though, because scratching was too painful. All the nerve damage prevented me from relieving even a little itch. To this day, no one can touch my stomach or upper left side, including my arm, without causing nausea and a pain that can't be defined.

I can't scratch an itch from my elbow all the way up my arm, down around to my stomach, and back. As Charlie Brown from *Peanuts* would say, "Ughh!" For more than two years, I couldn't wear jeans or anything that had a button, or put any kind of pressure on my stomach—the sensitivity from having all the nerve endings cut made it too painful.

I could wear only stretchy pants, and we all know how attractive those are. The only time you can get away with stretchy pants is during pregnancy. Then you have a really good excuse, but it's still tough to pull off. Even Cindy Crawford might not get away with that. Bald and wearing stretchy pants—not a great combo.

As colder weather settled in, I wore a puffy down coat because I was always so cold. I looked like a brown Michelin man. With stretchy black maternity pants, a red wig, a big brown hat with a little chemo cap underneath, no eyelashes or eyebrows, deep, dark circles under my eyes, and gray skin, I didn't even recognize myself.

I had wasted away to nothing. I felt horrible and looked horrible—and felt even more horrible because I looked horrible. I hope this doesn't come across as offensive, but the only way I can describe my appearance was to compare myself to pictures I had seen of war prisoners. Was that the best that modern medicine could do? There had to be a better way.

There were some small pleasures, such as going to a certain restaurant. But realistically, even the best food never tasted good once I started chemo. The tortellini at one Italian restaurant and the shakes at Serendipity—I was careful not to eat any of my favorites after one bad experience. I ordered one of my favorites: an Italian dish that was basically pot roast. I got so sick, I never wanted to eat or smell that or pot roast again. And I never did.

I was trapped in a nightmare. I was in an Edgar suit like Vincent D'Onofrio's in *Men in Black.* He was the alien who had been eaten by bugs.

When they unzipped his body, out came the alien. His wife sat on the couch explaining that it wasn't her husband. She kept saying, "It was an Edgar suit; he was in an Edgar suit." Then she shortened it to "Egger suit." Then she realized how funny it sounded, and laughed hysterically.

I was trapped inside an Egger suit. I was in someone else's body. *Somebody please unzip this thing and let me out!* Somewhere along the way, I'd lost my body.

Slowly, things began to turn around. I felt like it was time to put it all past me and move on with my life. That's when I lost my job after fourteen years, and with that went my life insurance, medical insurance, and disability insurance, too. I'd thought being told I couldn't have more children was worse than being told I had cancer, which it was. But this was my other baby. The day I lost my job was the day I lost hope.

It couldn't get any worse—that is, until my husband found a lump of his own.

Chapter Eight

IT'S A THUNDERSTORM:
KEVIN'S CANCER

There are those days when you receive certain kinds of news. You'll never forget where you were or what you were doing. Good news or bad. You never forget that moment or the details around you when you heard it. Like the day you were thrilled to discover you were finally pregnant, or when you learned of the devastation of Nine-eleven, or John F. Kennedy's assassination.

Our moment came over a pay phone in a hot, stinky train station, in a remote southern Italian town where no one spoke English. The train strike we had been caught in wasn't all that serious—unless, of course, you've just gotten a piece of very bad news.

Train strikes happen in Italy as often as we change our clothes in the States. Don't get me wrong. We absolutely *love* Italy. Given the opportunity, I would probably move there. But we're talking about life-changing moments. In that stinky, hot train station where no one spoke English, in the middle of a train strike, was where we found out Kevin had cancer.

Is there any way to describe the force you are hit with when the words "you have cancer" enter your energy field? Any way to describe that instantaneous shattering of your world with that unshakable knowledge that you could die? The only question was how long it would take.

It's the loss of innocence. It's no longer feeling immortal. Someone doesn't actually pound you in the stomach with a brick, but the energetic impact is about the same. This is followed almost instantaneously by the question "Can I live?"

Let's go back to the moments leading up to the stinky, hot train station. Kevin was in the shower when he felt a lump in his groin. At this point, we knew that our bodies were not meant to have lumps popping up in strange places. Actually, lumps weren't supposed to pop up *anywhere*. There were no usual places for lumps (except, of course, on a woman's chest).

"Obviously, it can't be anything," I reassured him. "That would just be ridiculous. You should go to the doctor anyway."

So he went. The doctor said he thought maybe Kevin banged into something at work. He did actually bang up his body quite a bit—an occupational hazard that came with building power plants. The doctor told him to come back in a month if it didn't get better.

A month later, he went back. The lump seemed to have gotten larger. The doctor suggested a sonogram.

"We're leaving in a few days for Italy," we said.

"Okay, so do it when you get back."

"Hey, Doc, I know a little too much about lumps to think there's no rush," I said. "We can't wait a couple of weeks to take care of this. I want him to have it biopsied before we go."

The marathon began. We had three days to have all the testing and surgery done.

"I'm sure it's nothing," the doctor said.

When have I heard that before? "Great. Let's do it anyway."

The biopsy was scheduled to take half an hour. The doctor would find me in the waiting room to let me know how it went.

In a half-hour procedure, it's never good when an hour, then an hour and a half, goes by with no word. But I remained optimistic. Finally the doctor called me.

"He's doing well. We removed the lump and will send it out to be biopsied. We should have the results in about a week."

"Okay, great. So does it seem like it's all right?"

"We'll just have to hope for the best."

WHAM!

"What? What's that supposed to mean?"

At first he didn't answer. Then, very solemnly, he said, "It means we just have to hope for the best."

I didn't have the heart to tell Kevin.

My mom had suggested that we go to Italy to see my aunt El and her husband, Toto, both of whom I adored. We could also make a pilgrimage to Pietrelcina to Padre Pio's shrine. He was a soon-to-be-anointed saint known to have performed many miracles, and God knew we could use one right about now. Maybe he could help us. After the AVM, my round of cancer, losing my job and Kevin discovering a lump, we could use all the help we could get. Besides, we missed Aunt El and Toto. And the trip would be easy and inexpensive, because we could use miles for the tickets and could stay with them.

Aunt El was one of those people with such a great spirit, you just wanted to tuck her under your arm and carry her around with you. She wasn't my blood aunt, but we were so close, she might as well have been. I loved spending time talking with her. She was brilliant and well read and could discuss just about anything.

She told the most romantic story of how she had ended up in Italy. She and my mom had been best friends since kindergarten, so that would be fifty-nine years. They had lived around the block from each other in Queens. They were inseparable—until one summer, when Aunt El went back to Italy to see her family.

Her parents had come from Italy to the States to create a better life for themselves, and they often went back home to visit. That particular summer, they went to Stromboli, a volcanic island off the coast of Sicily. There, at age fourteen, El met Toto, Ingrid Bergman, and Roberto Rossellini. Toto was irresistible—and still was, all these years later.

At eighteen, El went back and met him again, and that was it. They fell in love, and she moved to Italy. Fortunately, she and my mom stayed friends. We had gone to see her every few years. She wasn't able to travel much, because of a degenerative bone disease called osteogenesis imperfecta. It is also known as "glass (or brittle) bone disease," because the bones break very easily, even from sneezing or a simple fall. Despite that, El had made it back to the States a few years ago.

Aunt El and Toto had not yet met Kelsey, who was twenty months old by now. Mom, Kevin, Kelsey, and I arrived at the airport. Kelsey, who never allowed anyone new to carry her without screaming bloody murder, was scooped up into Toto's arms. He simply walked away with her, flashing his customs badge to all the officials so we could exit easily. She put her arm around his neck as if she had known him her whole life. That's just how irresistible and charismatic he was.

We spent the next few days visiting with our "cousins," Aunt El's children, Joey, Giovanna, and Enzo, whom I've known all my life, along with their families. We prayed at the Vatican, the Sistine Chapel, and the quaint old town of Marino. A strawberry festival was going on in the medieval town of Nemi, one of our favorites. We sipped wine in Friscati, and Mom and Kevin tested gelato everywhere they could find it. All lovely experiences, yet this cloud hung over us. I really wanted to get to San Giovanni Rotondo to see Padre Pio.

Well, okay, no one actually *sees* Padre Pio, since he passed away about forty years ago. But visitors go to a shrine to his memory. I first heard of him from my friend Joanne. It was right after I was diagnosed the first time. A lovely couple, Anna and Gino, were at Joanne's home and gave me a novena booklet and a piece of fabric. I was skeptical, but they seemed awfully nice, and Anna had had her own experiences meeting Padre Pio in person when Anna lived near him in Italy.

I call him "Padre" because that was how he was first introduced to me. He has since been named a saint by the Catholic Church, so he is Saint Pio. (I hope he doesn't mind that I still call him Padre Pio instead of Saint Pio!)

Anyway, Anna and Gino were devout Catholics and devotees of Padre Pio. They explained that Padre Pio had many proven miracles. One he hadn't been so thrilled to receive was the stigmata: wounds through his hands and feet, like the ones Jesus experienced during his crucifixion.

Although a wonderful honor, it was horribly painful. It also brought much chastising from the Catholic Church, which didn't accept the miracle. Padre Pio himself wanted nothing to do with it. However, the Church, after torturing him with scientific tests, finally agreed that he did in fact have the stigmata.

He lived a life of pain, but he also had many gifts. He had the ability to bilocate, which meant he could be in two places at the same time. He was proved to have said mass in two different cities at the same time. He had the ability to read a person's thoughts and would tell visitors to leave the confessional until they were willing to tell the whole truth. He sent them away with the specifics of what they had left out!

Most importantly, he had the ability to heal. You can believe this or not—it's really not relevant to understanding what happened for Kevin and me. I myself was skeptical, but given my limited options, I was willing to try anything. I share this for those who might believe. Believing you will be healed is vitally important to actually being healed. I also think it's important to tell you why we feel Padre Pio was part of our miracle, or at the very least a guide to our healing path.

The piece of fabric that Anna and Gino gave me was a tiny piece of one of Padre Pio's gloves. I pinned the fabric inside my bra on the side where I'd had the mastectomy. From that moment on, I repeated the Prayer of Padre Pio, asking Jesus, Mary, and God to help us.

I wasn't praying just for myself; I was praying for a lot of other people. Amazingly, whatever I prayed for came true. A friend of the family was having a "triple A," a serious operation to repair an abdominal aortic aneurism. His wish was for a fast recovery, and so I prayed very hard for him. The doctors were amazed by how quickly he recovered—the fastest ever, they said.

The stories went on and on. So this was the beginning of my belief in Padre Pio. I also think he wanted me to be less skeptical before I visited his shrine myself. So I made a pilgrimage to San Giovanni Rotondo. I felt such a strong pull, there was no question that I had to go there. The town was in the mountains in a remote part of Italy. We had no idea what we were getting into, but I took it on blind faith that I was meant to go.

✳   ✳   ✳

We prepared to leave for San Giovanni Rotondo. We had to leave at six in the morning, so Mom had us up at five. She and Kevin kept yelling at me to hurry. Kevin was always a wreck on a traveling day. He liked to be at the airport four hours ahead of time, while I preferred to do the OJ Simpson through the airport, jumping over luggage. Adding that to Kevin's discomfort didn't make for a good combination.

Anyway, we left at exactly six o'clock. I was feeling really proud of myself until I realized I'd forgotten my jacket. Since I was always cold, there was no question that I would go back for it. That went over really well. Kevin asked if I was chewing on a piece of gum. When I shook my head, he said, "Good. I was concerned you might be walking and chewing gum at the same time."

Nice. I stuck out my tongue. Very mature. I was getting a really bad rep. I was so exhausted, I couldn't believe I could walk at all. Kevin was right: better not to try chewing gum!

Aunt El accompanied us to the *termini,* the train station. She wasn't able to go with us, because it was too unsafe given her "glass bone" condition.

Kelsey had her first metro ride. She was amazed by how the doors opened and closed. We had to go up and down escalators and endless flights of stairs. Not great for Kevin or me, especially toting a stroller. The train would take us to Foggia, the main town nearest San Giovanni Rotondo.

We traveled second-class on a superstar train, like the Amtrak Bullet, with four seats facing each other. I couldn't wait to sleep. I prayed Kelsey would nap. She would have no part of sleeping, and whined and laughed at the same time. This was an adventure for her. At the second stop, a large group of young Italian men filled the train.

I had taken beginner Italian three times through a local continuing education program. Each time, something (pregnancy, for instance, and cancer) had happened to prevent me from moving on to the next level. So I had a pretty good grasp of a lot of useless information. I knew how to ask questions but couldn't really understand the answers. I loved this beautiful, romantic language and still plan on becoming fluent one day.

The mothers and girlfriends of these men were sobbing and hugging each other. The young men were traveling to the military base near Bari in the south of Italy. Most of them didn't seem old enough to have girlfriends, let alone be in the military. They were really loud, and I thought, *Oh, God, Kelsey and I are never going to be able to sleep.*

A few of them sat next to a very nice lady, and they turned out to be really sweet. They began playing with Kelsey and made her laugh, whistling at her and calling her name. They kept calling her "Chelsea," "*la figlia del suo presidente*"—"the daughter of your president" (Chelsea Clinton). Close enough.

Kevin answered, *"Un, me nombre Kevin,"* which is pretty much just butchered Spanish, not Italian, and means, "One, to me name Kevin."

He thought they were asking how many children he had and what his name was. He can be very cute. They must have thought, *silly American.* Kevin asked in English if they were military.

One said, *"Si, tutti,"* and swept his arm to indicate the entire train.

When it was time to get off, we said, *"Ciao!"* and Kelsey blew kisses. An old man started talking to me at the exit. Because I had carried on a quasi conversation with the soldiers, he assumed I spoke Italian. I sure fooled him. He was speaking too quickly, so I told him I only spoke a little Italian. I used one of my favorite phrases: *"Può parlare più lentamente, per favore?"* —roughly, "Can you speak more slowly, please?" I was shocked and excited when he understood me!

In Foggia, we went to the Office of Information, which is full of information that you can understand only if you speak Italian. Otherwise, it's the Office of No Information. We wanted to find out how to get to San Giovanni Rotondo. I just love saying "San Giovanni Rotondo" with my trying-to-sound-Italian accent while rolling the "R."

No one in the entire station spoke English. Aunt El had thought there would be plenty of people who could speak English—they must have been on strike. Out came my little Berlitz book, and I was able to buy the tickets for the bus.

Unfortunately, *finding* the bus was another story. One woman was kind enough to come out of the booth and point to where the bus was parked. I had no idea what she meant. I couldn't catch a word. There were three different lanes in the street, with islands in between. I had no idea what she meant until she said, *"Seduto."* Aha! That meant "seated." Yes, I saw it. People were seated. I was so excited to have understood, I tried to hug her. She jumped back. Sorry!

The bus ride took a terrifying, treacherous hour. Our destination was way, way up at the top of a mountain. We drove along cliffs, sometimes with only a single lane. Oh, my God, what had I done? What had I gotten us all into? This was not the way I want to go. Then again, cancer sucked as a way to go, too.

Next we had to find someone to tell us which stop was ours. A woman and a man who looked kind of creepy tried to help us. I felt a little uncomfortable, but beggars can't be choosers. We got off at the bottom of a hill. We had planned on searching for the hotel first.

Until we saw it. At the top of the hill, a massive picture of Padre Pio hung in front of the church. It took up half the facade. Once I saw that picture with that sweet face, I welled up with tears. I was really here! I couldn't stop crying. I had asked for his help and had told him I knew he would help us. I couldn't go straight to the hotel. He was the reason we had come, and I needed to go in right that minute to pray.

The only thing between him and me was the hill, which looked to be at a forty-five-degree slope. Kelsey lounged comfortably in her stroller with one leg hanging over the side, as if to say, "I belong here in San Giovanni Rotondo." Doesn't every twenty-month-old born to the O'Briens from Queens?

As we moved up the hill, the stroller took on weight—about a thousand pounds. When had this little pumpkin eaten all that pasta? Kevin was barely able to walk and winced with every step. Meanwhile, I was challenged just walking up a flight of steps, let alone a mountain. My mother ran circles around us. What a pair of misfits!

Zooming past Mom were the ninety-year-old ladies dressed head to toe in black, wearing high heels. I think one was about a hundred and twenty years old. It was a sad state of affairs for the O'Brien family. We prayed in front of Padre Pio's statue, and again downstairs in front of his tomb. I just kept crying and asking for his help. Also for God's, Mary's, Jesus's, Dad O'Brien's, and Mike's (the recently deceased father of my friend Joanne). We went back up to the main church to pray again.

I can only try to describe the power of what happened that day. I knelt in the pew with my mother and Kevin to my left. Kelsey was in the stroller on my right. Maybe five hundred people milled around inside the church—and not very reverently, I might add. They chattered away. I remember being a little annoyed that they didn't realize how special this place was. I had come all the way from New York to be here, yet they acted as though they were at the mall!

I began to pray to Padre Pio and God. The church had something mystical about it, a very special energy. I prayed with my eyes closed, probably more intensely than ever before. I entered what I can only describe as a "nothingness." Suddenly, everything went black. It was dead silent, and I was no longer aware of anything around me. There wasn't a single thought in my normally chatter-filled head.

As I stayed in this blackness, this dead silence, this nothingness, something indescribable occurred. A white ball of light headed straight at me. It hit me full force and filled my entire body, and an intense peace came over me. In that moment, I felt this was no ordinary light. It was divine. In my mind's eye, I placed Kevin in front of me. I scooped up the light that had penetrated my body, and pushed it toward him. Like a blast, it went straight to his leg, right where he had just had the surgery.

I was unaware of time or space in this nothingness, until a sound penetrated my bliss. It was very soft at first; then it got louder. It was a beautiful voice. It sounded familiar, but I was still partly in a trance. With no other sound in the church, I again heard "Papa. Papa."

That beautiful, angelic voice repeated, "Papa. Papa." I slowly opened my eyes and adjusted to the light as I turned to the voice. Kelsey was staring up at the ceiling, toward the center of the church, with a sweet little smile. She was saying, "Papa, Papa," as if she recognized someone and wanted us to say hello, too. She couldn't take her eyes off the ceiling.

I took in the immensity of what had just happened. Things like that just didn't happen in my life. I had never before had that experience of darkness and silence and divine light. I could only pray to be blessed enough to experience that again—to get back to that depth of peace, a knowingness of something so much greater than my current existence.

As Kelsey uttered, "Papa, Papa"—a word she had never said before—Kevin and I looked at each other. He was perplexed, but I smiled. What had she seen while that light filled me? Which "papa" had she seen, God the Father, or Padre Pio the father? I don't know, but she saw something. Something tremendously powerful happened in that church on top of that mountain.

Chapter Nine

MALIGNANT MELANOMA

The steep hills were very hard on us. The hotel was at the bottom, and the church at the top. Kevin's leg grew worse after we left the church. The golf ball at the base of the incision had grown, and he was as concerned as I was. I wanted him to go to the hospital.

The hospital, conveniently located next to the church, was called *Casa sollievo della sofferenza*—"home for relief of the suffering." "Relief of the suffering" sounded like a good idea to me. Everything sounded better in Italian. Even suffering didn't sound so bad. However, the man who didn't want to cause any fuss, the man who downplayed everything, wanted to wait.

The hotel was lovely—much nicer than we had anticipated. It was really more like a convent run by nuns. We felt very welcome, and meals were included! It had been hard for Aunt El to send us off to San Giovanni Rotondo on our own, as if it were our first day of kindergarten. She had already left a message to call as soon as we got in, but the nuns whisked us off to the dining room to make sure we ate before lunch was over.

Five minutes later, Aunt El phoned again. Poor thing, she was frantic with worry. Since we had gone to the church first, we were pretty late connecting with her. It was so sweet. She had really wanted to come along, but it was just too dangerous for her. We ate and had our afternoon siesta.

Kevin's leg turned much worse. It grew burning hot, as if it were on fire. It took me a good thirty minutes to get the nuns to understand that we needed ice. He still didn't want to go to the hospital. When would I ever learn not to listen to him? He wanted us to go on to mass without him. The six o'clock mass was packed. I caught only a couple of words. Kelsey was an angel again. She played with her shoelaces and her Travel Magna Doodle, then had a ball running around outside.

Kevin joined us again, and we enjoyed a cappuccino on the veranda of the hotel while Kelsey ran around rearranging the chairs. It was great to share her joy, even though my insides twisted with sheer terror at the thought of what we might hear tomorrow. I continued praying for our miracle. I still felt that everything would be okay eventually.

The next day was not as good. Actually, it turned into the day from hell. Instead of one golf ball, Kevin now had two, spread wide apart, and they were getting big enough that we actually could have putted them like golf balls.

We wanted to catch the nine o'clock mass before heading back to Rome. None of us were in the best of states, including Kelsey. Until now she had been wonderful, so we had to expect a bad day. She was exhausted and lasted only a few minutes in church this time. I had myself, Kelsey, Kevin, Mom, my two rosary beads, and the angel pin I wore inside my bra all blessed. We also had pictures of my nieces and nephews blessed.

Kevin and I were completely exhausted, and Kelsey wore us down further. I felt as if I had nothing left. Now we had to wait for the bus back down the mountain. When the church bells rang, Kelsey stopped running around. She looked so reverent putting her little hands together in prayer until the bells stopped and then started running around again. I've always called her my precious little angel and God's blessing. There has always been something very special about her, as if she has some kind of powerful connection.

So we waited. And waited. Was there a bus strike, too? In Italy, you never knew. The bus that finally arrived was hot and rickety, and we wondered if the wheels would fall off as we headed down the mountain. There was no air conditioning, which added to our misery. Kelsey never took heat well. She got beet red and boiling hot, looking like a real tomato-head.

Aunt El told us to check with the clerk at the front desk of the hotel before we left, to make sure there wasn't a train strike. The clerk assured us there wasn't. She was wrong. After the treacherous ride down the mountain, without an ounce of energy left, we arrived at the station to discover that there was, in fact, a strike. Did I mention that not a single soul spoke English?

I showed my ticket to the man in the information booth. With my little smattering of Italian, I understood him to say we could use it for the train at 7:20 p.m. Why they would have a strike for eight hours was beyond me. Why bother?

It was only noon, so we had quite a wait in the hot, smelly station. We wondered how—and if—we would get home and whether there would actually be a train at 7:20. It didn't seem to bother the Italians one bit. No one seemed remotely upset. It was business as usual. But if you hadn't traveled thousands of miles by car, train, plane, and bus with two mutating golf balls on your leg while waiting to hear whether you were going to die, you might not be so uptight, either.

So we waited. We waited for the train strike to be over. We waited for someone who could speak English. We waited for the doctor's office in New York to open—four hours for that. Sheer torture. We tried to rent a car, but they had only stick shifts. We tried to take a plane but missed the only flight to Rome. So we had to stick it out in this sweaty, funky-smelling train station.

I couldn't imagine making that call from a pay phone. What were the odds of a train strike today? Pretty good, actually. The worst part was the wait. Always the wait. I really didn't want to call the doctor, because I knew it was bad news. Worse, I knew more than Kevin. He wasn't the least bit prepared. But he would have gone into a deep depression if I'd said anything earlier.

I probably shouldn't have kept it from him. But he would have been so much more miserable if he had known. Wouldn't he? Okay, I sucked it up and admitted I had no right to keep it from him.

So we waited … tick, tick, tick … I realized why one woman in the surgeon's office hadn't been in a rush to get the results of a biopsy. Now I knew why she had said, "I'd rather have a little more time in oblivion. Reality is something I don't want to face."

Isn't it strange how a stranger can leave such a lasting impression on you? She had polled a bunch of people who were diagnosed with cancer, and discovered they all had experienced some trauma or exceptional stress two years before their diagnoses. She had lost her son. Another woman had gotten divorced.

I did the math. Two years before I was diagnosed, Kevin had the brain hemorrhage. Two years before our wait in the train station, the doctors thought Kelsey had spina bifida. Maybe there *was* something to her theory.

The other thing she said was that she had been diagnosed five years before. She had been so enraged by her cancer that if anyone in the waiting room laughed, she felt like jumping across the room and ripping their head off. I couldn't say I'd ever felt that way. If I saw someone laughing, I also wanted to be in on the joke. I really could have used something to laugh about!

That was exactly how I felt sitting in the train station. I could really use something to laugh about. Even the Italians weren't laughing, and they were *always* laughing. They weren't throwing things, but they weren't laughing, either. That didn't seem right.

Finally, four o'clock rolled around. I waited until one minute after. I was grateful to be able to figure out how to use the phone card. Kevin was understandably uptight. I could have waited a year to call, because I didn't want to hear the inevitable. If the doctor had good news, he would have called or e-mailed. But maybe he was really, really busy and hadn't gotten around to it.

The phone rang. They put me right through. As soon as I heard the tone of the doctor's voice, I knew. It was that *I'm really sorry* tone. The news was worse than we had expected: malignant melanoma—an especially aggressive form of cancer.

*   *   *

It doesn't matter whether you're prepared. Even if you think you already know the verdict, no one's ready to actually hear the words. I was still dealing with side effects from my own trial, and suddenly Kevin had cancer. He was only thirty-four. It was unthinkable.

I did what I could to be strong, but it knocked the wind out of me. I had trouble breathing. I couldn't finish the conversation with the doctor without choking on my sobs. I had to stop breathing. I stopped talking and waited. I waited until I could breathe without crying. Then I waited until I could *speak* without crying.

I looked at Kevin. He knew. His eyes welled up. I looked at Kelsey. How could this be? I couldn't imagine our beautiful angel without parents. You can't keep those thoughts from breaking in. Who would raise her? Would not having parents destroy her beautiful spirit?

I looked at my mom. How much more could she bear? She had lived her life for us for three years. How much more could *she* take? Her eyes welled up. She knew without my having to say a word.

I am so sorry, Kevin, I thought. *I am just so sorry.*

He held me as we cried. We walked around in shock for a while. Minutes? Hours? Who could tell anymore? We were in this hot, god-awful train station, and Kevin had cancer. And we had to wait here for three more hours—*if* we were lucky and the train strike really ended by then.

Kevin hugged Kelsey and held her tight. I had to turn away. I couldn't hold back anymore. It was ridiculous even to try. I completely broke down. Not a delicate breaking down, but an embarrassing, sobbing, snot-running-down-my-face-that-I-wiped-with-my-arms breaking down. I was terrified. I just didn't understand.

Mom tried to console me, but she lost it, too. She told me to be strong, and I knew I had to be, but every time I looked at Kevin and Kelsey, I started crying again. They loved each other so much. He was such an awesome dad. My heart broke at how scared he must be. He was thinking the worst, and I wasn't thinking any differently.

Finally, he said, "I'm afraid it's already in the major organs."

"We'll get the best doctors," I said. "We'll get you better no matter what it takes."

It was the only thing I could say. My heart sank at his next words.

"I prayed that Padre Pio would make me better," he said. "I also prayed that if God has to take one of us, it should be me. You'll make a better single parent."

That he could even think that way hit me like a cannonball to the gut. *He amazes me,* I thought. *I love him.* He had the biggest heart in the world. I'd felt the same way when I was diagnosed: that he would make a better parent if God should take me. But I'd never prayed for God to take me instead of him. I was selfish—I wanted us both to live.

I couldn't stomach the thought that Kelsey might lose both of us. This precious little angel not having parents on her wedding day or during the birth of her first child … I couldn't breathe. The thoughts sucked the life out of me. I knew, though, that I couldn't keep letting Kevin see me cry. He had this sweet look on his face and told me not to cry. How could he look at me like that and tell me not to cry?

The next best thing to letting it out by crying was to go into action. If I was going to make things happen, we had to work toward making Kevin better. I called the travel agent in New York to ask her to start the insurance paperwork and whatever else we needed for an emergency return. I asked my oncologist to find the absolutely best melanoma doctor at the hospital. When I told Aunt El, she was a wreck, speechless. We asked her to get in touch with the airline and change the tickets so we could return to the States as soon as possible.

The rest of the trip was brutal. An already horrible situation became absolutely horrific. Kelsey was unbearable. She was exhausted, but she wouldn't sleep. When the train finally arrived, we had to squeeze into the packed car and were separated. The conductor had the nerve to tell Kevin he was on the wrong train and needed to get off.

The nerve! Kevin found out he had cancer, and because this guy was on strike, we couldn't get back to Rome. Mom and I were trying to calm Kelsey down at that moment. Otherwise I would have climbed over all those people and ripped that conductor's head off—just as that lady in the doctor's office had said she wanted to do when people laughed.

I was done, just completely done. There was nothing left.

After finally getting back to Rome at one in the morning, we cried with Aunt El for what seemed like hours. We left the next morning. So long, Italy. Sorry we couldn't stay a little longer.

We expected to hit the ground running. After all, we were already pros at cancer. Since Kevin's tumor had already been removed, we were ready to start the chemo. We didn't hit the ground running, though—all the running did was bang us right into walls.

The doctor said, "Before we can discuss any treatment, you have to have more surgery and tests. First we have to remove the rest of the surrounding lymph nodes to see how far it's traveled."

The first lump, which had been a lymph node, had been entirely overtaken by cancer, which had likely spread to other lymph nodes. Given how aggressive this type of cancer was and how large the tumor had been, we were prepared for it to be in his organs.

Another surgery. What could we do about that? Find the best surgeon specializing in melanoma, that's what. Kevin had a second surgery, followed by more days in the hospital. He was depressed and angry. In his mind, he was already dead.

Another week waiting for the results. Why did we have to wait so long for biopsy results? How was it that later, when my surgeon knew she had screwed up, she had been able to get the results back in hours? Why must we be tortured with waiting? I couldn't help but wonder if it was all to protect doctors—and their insurers—against lawsuits. Did *their* parents, sisters, wives, or children have to wait a week? Could someone please explain this?

On the bright side, imagine everyone's surprise when the results showed no cancer in the other lymph nodes. I thought back to that experience in the church, when I watched the light shoot into Kevin's leg. I wondered how no signs of cancer could show up in the other lymph nodes when the one they removed had been stuffed full. Do you wonder, too?

Kevin did have a spot on his lung, though, and another on his shin. They could biopsy the shin, but it was too difficult to biopsy the lung, given the location of the spot. They would just have to watch it. The results of the testing indicated stage 3b, possibly stage 4, but they couldn't confirm without the biopsy. They also couldn't find a primary site where the melanoma had started, so they had no idea if it was a distant metastasis, which would be worse.

Being optimistic, I said it was 3b. That was my story, and I was sticking to it. Kevin's chances of survival were between 20 and 30 percent.

That really sucked. The next six months were hell in a way that was all-consuming, like being on a burning plane spiraling to earth.

As it turned out, the surgery and the spot on the lung weren't the worst of it. Two other things were. First, melanoma was a very hard cancer to treat. There really wasn't much they could do. There wasn't any effective conventional treatment. The disease was extremely aggressive and didn't respond to chemotherapy. Wasn't it bad enough that we both had cancer? He had to have the kind that didn't respond to chemo.

The second? The only suggested treatment, interferon, often made the patient want death instead. But by now, you know I don't usually take the first answer if I don't like it. Kevin would say that was pretty typical for our relationship. In a way, I was like a little kid—I would just keep pushing and pushing until I got that candy bar. Usually, my focus was on something silly; now it was on my husband's life.

After searching for a couple of weeks for trials, we found very few. In fact, we found only one. It was a two-year study with two control groups. One group got interferon plus a trial vaccine; the other got interferon plus a placebo.

It was all we had, and it was being done right here in good old New York City. We met with the doctor, did a whole bunch of testing, and were accepted. It meant weekly trips into the city and being monitored for two years. During the trial, Kevin would inject himself in the stomach with interferon. The side effects were flulike symptoms that "hung around a month or two."

Once again, nothing prepared the patient for what that actually meant. Most of us have had the flu. You have it for a day or two, maybe three days if it's really bad. But who can appreciate what it would be like to have the flu for a month or two with no reprieve? And not just an ordinary flu—the worst case imaginable.

And so it began. My big, strapping guy was completely broken. Kevin was so sick, he couldn't get out of bed. He had constant fevers of 104. I'll never forget how I walked into the bedroom after he started the injections, and he was shaking so violently, I had to lie on top of him to hold him down and try to warm him up.

He was so cold, he needed my body heat and all the extra blankets I could find, and still he wasn't warm. Then came the headaches, fatigue, depression and manic behavior, insomnia, racing thoughts, anger and just all-around messed-up stuff. His mood changes were frightening.

It was as if a switch had flipped in his brain, starting back when he had the brain hemorrhage. Something in his brain changed then, and was activated in full force when he started the treatments. He would just snap. He became a different person: manic one minute, depressed the next, and lunatic the next. It was horrible.

Then came a full-body PET scan to see if there was cancer anywhere else. It showed a significant hot spot in the ankle bone, which concerned the doctors quite a bit. He needed more surgery for a biopsy. Dear God, when was this going to end?

*　　*　　*

We found out that there was also a shrine for Padre Pio in Pennsylvania. We just had to go. The trip took about three hours by car. We met the most loving, caring, wonderful people there, including Vera Calandra's daughter. Vera had established the shrine after her daughter experienced a miraculous healing with Padre Pio.

When they heard about my experience in San Giovanni Rotondo, one of them whispered that they had Padre Pio's actual glove at the shrine. They kept it locked away, but when we explained what was going on, one of these wonderful women got it out. They held it to Kevin's heart and his ankle while praying fervently.

I felt such peace come over me. It was going to be okay. I was still terrified, of course, and constantly had that ping-pong match going in my head and heart. But each time I finally calmed down, I kept coming back to *It's going to be okay.*

What happened next was another of those moments that either you believe or you don't. Kevin was scheduled for surgery to biopsy his ankle with one of New York's top orthopedic cancer surgeons. He was having a hard time with all this. We waited again through those torturous hours of surgery for the doctor to come out. Was it in his bones? That would be the worst possible scenario. After several hours, the doctor visited my mother, my sister Kathy, and me.

"Well," he said, "I really can't explain what I found. There doesn't appear to be any cancer, but the bone had an unusual consistency I can't really describe. It was mushy, as if something had eaten away at it, but there doesn't appear to be any cancer. I haven't seen anything like this before."

My mouth dropped open. He continued in a professional tone, unaware of the significance of his words.

"I removed a significant amount of the deteriorated bone, so his ankle is in danger of snapping easily. We'll put a cast on to protect it. He'll probably be in quite a bit of pain for a while and will have to be very careful walking."

I believed we had just received another unexplainable miracle. What do you think?

As we went back to the trial group each week, one patient after another had recurrences. We grew more terrified. Young people, even younger than Kevin, were dying. One week, we showed up at the hospital to discover that the trial had been canceled—they weren't even allowing people to continue with the interferon.

"The trial just was not effective," Kevin's oncologist said. "I'm sorry."

"Can't they let us keep doing it?" Kevin asked. "I mean, come on. There's nothing else out there, nothing else we can do."

Even if it didn't work, at least we were doing something. Hope alone was enough reason to continue.

"Nope. Sorry, guys."

That was it. Party over.

"Okay, God," I said, "now what? I'm not hearing you loud and clear. What are we supposed to do? You know I need you to hit me over the head."

So what did we do? We moved on. We got back to life—life without cancer.

Chapter Ten

THE TYPHOON: STAGE 4

Phew! Glad that whole cancer thing was over.

After searching for eighteen months, I finally got a new job. Kevin returned to work, and we had a huge luau to celebrate getting back to life. Over a hundred and twenty friends and family came. With 87 percent odds of remaining cancer free, I was golden. We were going to live it up.

Before I started my new job, we went to my cousin Michael's wedding in Bermuda. Maybe the best wedding, best trip, I had ever experienced, trapped on that beautiful island for five days, no kids, and loads and loads of fun. After the long, lovely weekend was over, we flew back to JFK, where I said good-bye to Kevin and hopped on another plane to meet my family for a long-anticipated, much-prepared-for tour of London, Paris, and Rome.

Yes, Rome. I would get to speak Italian! Yahoo! I even went back to say hi to Padre Pio. So what if we went into debt. Who knows—I could get hit by a truck tomorrow, right? Actually, my mom had been saving to take us on this trip for years. It had long been a dream of hers.

At this point, I began to be grateful. Yes, that's right, I was feeling pretty blessed. When I looked back on my bout with cancer, I thought, *Wow, I was lucky it was just me who had it at the time.* So I chose to feel blessed. And Kelsey was our greatest blessing. I had an opportunity to spend more time with her. We were also blessed with family and friends willing to pitch in and help with anything at the drop of a hat. We had so much support, with my mom the angel leading the charge. Without her help, we would have been lost.

This is the lesson I learned and that I want to share: be happy with what you have right now. There will always be someone else worse off, and things could always be worse. If I had thought it couldn't get worse, nothing could have prepared me for what happened next.

If you put your arms up and ask for what you need, you'll get it. Well, I must have been praying for a brick to fall on my head.

Actually, it was more like a tidal wave—that was the day I learned that I was going to die.

Did God make some kind of mistake? Maybe it was a practical joke. Had he been off on a siesta somewhere and not noticed that he had already given us more than enough to handle?

"You *are* kidding, right?" I said, laughing, to no one in particular.

It really *was* laughable—that is, of course, if you're the one going through it. I was the only one who could laugh about it, because everyone else was so shocked and horrified, they didn't know how to pick their jaw up off the floor, let alone pull out the right thing to say.

If it happens to someone you know, don't worry about it—there's really nothing you *can* say. Just don't say, "I'm sorry." It's natural enough, but don't do it. You can say, "That sucks, man," or "That's messed up, dude [or dudette]." Or "They must have made a mistake," or "Come on, let's go get drunk," or "I heard really athletic sex is good for taking the edge off situations like this."

Okay, maybe don't use that last one.

Whatever you do, though, don't say, "I'm sorry." To me, that meant you had already agreed that I was going to die.

*   *   *

I had recently started my new job. Given that I had worked in a very specialized area of the brokerage community, it was hard to find an employer who couldn't pick up the phone and find out I'd had cancer. Who wanted to risk hiring me? A friend of a friend, that's who, and I am eternally grateful to him and the owner of the company for seeing past that whole cancer thing and hiring me anyway.

I wound up getting two job offers the same week. They were both great opportunities, but the one I picked allowed me to work part of the week on Long Island and part in Manhattan. That meant a little more time with my daughter on the days when I didn't have to commute nearly four hours. Or so I thought. I wound up putting in a load of extra hours anyway.

Mom took Kelsey so Kevin and I could spend a weekend on the beach at Montauk. Two years had passed since I was diagnosed. The weather was beautiful—not warm enough to go in the water, but great for walks and breathing in that beautiful sea air.

We loved the sound of the waves crashing on the beach. Our dream was to own a beach house, where we could listen to the waves as we watched them break. The ocean was magnificent. It was majestic, powerful—something to be feared, yet peaceful and relaxing at the same time. It had so many emotions.

As we walked hand in hand along the sand, I casually mentioned that the lump I'd had for the past year seemed to have gotten bigger and harder. He stopped right there. Turning to me, he said, "You need to get it checked out."

"Well," I said naively, "I told Dr. X and Dr. Y about it this whole year, and they said it was nothing."

"You need to get it checked out," he said sharply.

"Okay, okay, I'll get it checked out."

That week, I saw the surgeon in Manhattan. She felt the lump and said, "It seems to be scar tissue, but we'll do a biopsy just to be sure."

I was fine, really. I didn't think it would be anything. My doctors had seemed so confident the whole year, telling me it was nothing. Of *course* I believed them. The surgeon would let me know in a couple of days.

The evening after the biopsy, I was a little drained from work and the long trip home from the city, and I was in pain from the biopsy. Around eight o'clock, just a few minutes after I walked in the door, the phone rang. It was Dr. Y. "Hi, Dr. Y," I said, chipper as can be, because I knew she wouldn't have the results for a few days. She must be calling to see how I felt after the biopsy.

"Joyce, the biopsy results came back," she said.

"Yes?"

"It's malignant."

Silence. I shook my head slowly. I looked at Kevin as tears filled my eyes. That wave hit me. You know, the real cruncher, the one that keeps you down so you can't breathe, can't speak, because you're too busy drowning.

"Malignant?" The whisper barely got past my lips. "I don't understand. You've been telling me for a year it was nothing to worry about. How can it be malignant?"

"I'm sorry."

I didn't want to hang up. There must be more to be said, but I couldn't think of anything. I was wide-eyed with shock and couldn't speak. I didn't know what this meant. It was not getting through to me yet.

"We'll have to do surgery to remove the mass."

Surgery? Oh, my God. No, I can't. I just can't do this again. No, God, please, not again. I can't do surgery again. I can't do cancer again. Please, no, not again.

I couldn't even cry. I'd just been punched in the chest. My lungs had collapsed. I couldn't do this again. I just couldn't. Oh, God, NO! My throat constricted. Kelsey was at my feet, looking up at me wide-eyed. She was three, and she knew something was wrong, terribly wrong. She seemed to know not to say anything. I leaned on the table and covered my face. I couldn't even cry. There were no more tears left. All that was left was shock.

I thought, *How am I going to tell Mom?*

And so it began. I sat in my office waiting for the oncologist to call. At least I knew what an oncologist was. Clearly, I was still the craziologist. It was about a quarter after eight in the evening, and I was finishing a project for work. I was trying to keep my mind occupied until I found out what the treatment would be—gathering data to figure out how to proceed with my life and work the treatment in at the same time.

The phone rang. I was eager because I wanted to get moving. You know, deal with it and move on again, as I had tried to do so many times already. I would have chemo, I was sure—lose my hair again, get really sick again. Would I be able to keep working?

Nothing, but *nothing* in this entire world could have prepared me for that call.

"Hi, Dr. X."

"Hi. How are you doing?"

"I'm okay." (A bit of an exaggeration.) "How are you?"

"Okay."

And you know I'm just being polite. I've always really liked you, but you misdiagnosed me for the past year and now I don't think I really like you all that much.

"I guess you've heard the biopsy was malignant," I said.

"Yes. It's the same cancer."

Here came the naive me, who thought she had this cancer thing down.

"Okay, that's good." Silence. "Isn't it?"

I was certain it was. After all, I'd had enough to deal with over the first one. I sure didn't want a whole new type … right?

"Actually, it's not good news. It's bad."

"Why is it bad?"

"Because it means the cancer has progressed. A new one might have meant it was at the beginning stages, so that would have been easier to stop."

"Oh . . ." I paused. "So will the chemo be the same as the last time?"

"Uh, no. You should come in so we can talk."

"No? Why not?"

"With a recurrence of this type, we won't do chemo."

"Okay. Radiation?"

"You should come in so we can talk about it."

"Dr. X, I'm not going to wait until I come in. I want to know right now what I need to do. I just want to know what type of treatment we have to do to cure it."

"I don't know that we'll be treating it at this time."

"What? How can we *not* treat it!"

"Joyce, it's stage 4. With stage four . . ."

"STAGE FOUR?"

I felt as if I were underwater and no words could get through, even though I knew that someone was talking. Everything choked up. I was going to throw up. My hand went to my mouth to keep me from letting out a horrible gasping sound, and I stifled a cry. I had a glass window looking into the hall, and anyone walking by could see.

"How can it be stage four!" I nearly shrieked. "What happened to stage three-a ... and three-b?"

"When you have a recurrence of the same cancer that has metastasized, it's stage four. Unfortunately, there's nothing we can do to cure you. All we can do is treat it as a chronic illness and give you as much time as possible."

As much time as possible? Oh, my God. I was only thirty-five, and my husband had cancer. I had a three-year-old child. Could it get any worse? She continued talking as if she couldn't hear the screaming inside my head.

"Studies show"—there we went again—"that chemo and radiation will not be able to cure you.

How could they not want to do any kind of treatment?

"Why don't you come in so we can talk about it?"

Talk about it—was she for real? How *could* we talk about it? I had told her something was wrong a year ago, nine months ago, six months ago, and three months ago. She had said it was nothing to worry about, and now she was saying she wouldn't treat it, because it was stage four and there wasn't anything she could do to save me.

I had always liked her as a person. But in that moment, I felt something I had rarely felt before: anger mixed with hatred and betrayal. I don't think I had ever hated anyone as long as I lived. But this was my *life* we were discussing. I felt as if my life had been taken away by her and the surgeon's lack of action.

"Please come in so we can talk."

"Yeah, sure, I'll come in," I replied. It was a Monday.

"I can see you Friday.

Friday! Was she kidding me? Because she had screwed up, I had stage 4 cancer, and she couldn't see me until *Friday*?

"I can't wait until Friday."

My head was spinning. I felt dizzy (it seemed to be happening a lot these days), my heart was pounding so hard I could barely breathe, and I didn't know what to do next.

"I'm sorry," she said. "I'm not available until Friday."

I wanted to run. Run away from my own life. This couldn't be my life. *Someone please wake me up, because I need to get off this ride.*

I had to call Kevin.

"Kevin, I just spoke to the doctor, and she said it's stage four and they aren't going to do any treatment, because it won't help. There's nothing they can do to save me."

"Oh, God. Oh, Joyce, I am so sorry."

I lost it. I had to get out of the office before anyone saw me like this. I sobbed the whole drive home. Thank God I hadn't taken the train today—that would have been ugly.

When I arrived, Kevin hugged me. He didn't say a word. He just hugged me as I cried. Kelsey looked up with that sweet little face. She was an old soul. She knew. I knelt down and pulled her into my arms. She put her chubby arms around me and patted me on the back as she said, "Grown-ups don't cry, Mommy."

This one has done more than her share, my sweet child.

I wanted to talk to their boss. They'd screwed this up pretty royally. I wanted to hear from him that there was nothing they could do.

Let's call him Dr. Coldheart.

You could tell that Dr. Coldheart had more important places to be and that I was an inconvenience. It was late Friday afternoon and he had places to go, people to see, and things to do. He reluctantly met with us. We could feel that he just wanted to get out of that office, and we were a nuisance.

He was as arrogant as anyone could be. I've worked with a lot of arrogant people on Wall Street, but to be that arrogant with someone's life, especially after the people who worked for you had screwed up … well, that was pretty arrogant.

"Stage four is stage four," he said. "It doesn't matter if we found it now or a year ago—the outcome is still the same. There's nothing we can do to save you. Studies show . . ."

Blah, blah, blah. Again, I know, vulgarity isn't very ladylike, and I wouldn't say this out loud, but there are some moments where no other word has the same impact, even if spoken only in my head.

F*** the studies! I screamed mentally. *I want to live! Give me something to work with here, dude.*

"So you're not going to treat me?" I was pleading for my life.

"That's right."

I felt that he was dismissing me and just wanted to be rid of me. That was it? Could he really be that flippant with my *life?* He was blatantly indifferent. I was a liability, no longer good for their statistics. Not even a simple "I'm sorry we screwed up and let this grow for a year even though you told us it was there." Or "Sorry your husband is sick and you have a three-year-old and we screwed up and didn't listen to you."

Come live a day in my life, Dr. Coldheart. Oh, wait. He did say one more thing.

"Is that all?" he asked. "I need to leave now. It *is* Friday night, and I *do* have other commitments."

The fact that Kevin was restrained enough not to grab him by his arrogant little neck and rip off his fat, arrogant head amazed me. The veins were visibly pumping in Kevin's neck. I secretly wished he would go ahead and punch our dear Dr. Coldheart's lights out.

I couldn't imagine having another surgery. The very thought made me sick to my stomach. I couldn't bear the thought of going through any more pain. Memories of the mastectomy flooded through me. I was terrified, horrified. It scared me more than I can put into words. I'd had all I could take. They had already cut many of the nerves in my abdomen, arm, and back. I still couldn't bear to have my skin touched. How could I handle another surgery?

There was a brief moment of bliss. As I was coming out of sleep, there was the moment spent half awake in twilight, in a place where everything was beautiful and peaceful and where I had a smile on my face. Then came the gut punch of fully waking up. It happened the moment I remembered the reality of my life. Now I know why people drink.

We had already planned a short trip to Disney World over Halloween weekend. My best friend, Diane, her husband, Curt, their children, and Curt's sisters and brothers-in-law were all going. No, we weren't Rockefellers. One of Curt's sisters, Pam, had a timeshare in a huge condo. They were so generous, they had saved up points for a long time so we could vacation together.

How do you go to Disney World when you've just been diagnosed with stage 4 cancer? The better question is, how do you *not* go? I mean, come on, I was probably in the worst emotional state of my life. What better place was there? The gnawing, sinking feeling never left my stomach, but Disney World with good friends, a bunch of screaming, happy kids, and a Halloween parade was a pretty good distraction.

After we got back, it was time for surgery. So I was wheeled into that same pre-op surgical room. Memory flooded over me again, and I choked up. I was sick at the thought of having to do it again. I didn't want to see or talk to anyone. I just wanted it to be over—no big hoopla, just over.

They removed the tumor, and I dealt with the pain. I was going to find a way to get better, because I was terrified of the pain of dying from cancer. I had known people who died of cancer, and all I could think of was the pain. I couldn't handle any more pain. At least this time, there were no biopsy results to wait for. They already knew it was cancer. Or so I thought.

I could never come up with this on my own. The writers of a movie couldn't think this one up. You really have to laugh because it was so ridiculous. She hadn't gotten "clean margins." She hadn't gotten all the cancer. It was already in my skin, the biggest organ of the body—I needed another surgery to remove more.

I know. *You're joking, right?*

There were also spots in my lung and neck, but there would be no more biopsies. Since that would have meant more surgery, I can't say I was unhappy about that decision.

No one knew what to say to us anymore. There were no words. People were mostly just silent. They were there for us in their silence. What could they have said? It was ridiculous even to try.

Chapter Eleven

THE RAIN IS LETTING UP: DEFINING MOMENTS

I'm sorry, I'm just not going to die.

That was it. I didn't care what Dr. Coldheart said; I wasn't going to die. I had a three-year-old, and a husband whose odds for hangin' with us much longer weren't so great. I wasn't going to die. I was going to find a way to live. It wasn't a matter of *if* I was going to do it. It was only a matter of *how*.

You might wonder how I got involved in the next stage of my journey. Someone who had never even been in a health food store, whose only experience with vitamins had been taking prenatals, or who popped one of her mom's Centrums once in a while. How did someone like me get involved in something that goes way beyond the scope of conventional thinking in the effort, ultimately, to save a life? Something—oh, no, don't say it!—something … *alternative*!

There, I said it. Glad you asked.

Now I'll share a defining moment. One of those moments when a much higher power intercedes—something so much bigger than we are, we often don't believe it's possible. We especially don't believe we are worthy of it happening to us.

You can call it God, the universe, a miracle, or whatever floats your boat. Either you believe or you don't. Either you take action or you don't. It's given to you. All you have to do is get past the fear and take action. Well, I had three such moments. How I had been so blessed, I'm not sure. I'm only now beginning to understand it.

I had always believed that out of every bad situation, something good can come. You just have to look for the good thing, which sometimes is nearly impossible to see in the moment. There's always some kind of life lesson. Maybe it's just a different way of thinking. Maybe someone does something really nice for you and it renews your faith in people. Maybe you renew a relationship because of it, or end a really harmful one. Or maybe you're guided in a way that alters your life permanently.

People often ask how I did it. How did I take this horrific situation and beat all the odds when there really wasn't any hope? How did I wind up going down this path? I tell them, "I dunno. I think God told me to look in the Yellow Pages." Seriously! I didn't get the message the first *two* times we had cancer, so I needed to be slammed with this brick.

God didn't actually speak to me. But some kind of divine guidance was certainly being offered. You know, when God closes a window, he opens a door. He didn't just open a door, though—he opened a whole universe. At the time, I couldn't think of a single good thing to come out of all we had been through, but when I looked hard I could usually find something. It really did help put me in a better place when the whole world seemed to be crumbling apart.

Let's go back two and a half years, to the spring before I was diagnosed the first time. Seems like an eternity, doesn't it? I had been promoted and had all those pregnancy-related basketballs hanging off my body for eight months. That left me a little, um, shall we say, awkwardly out of shape.

My body was out of shape in a way that didn't conform to conventional sizing, not to mention the cottage cheese my skin had turned into. Cellulite!

Anyway, I had been promoted to managing director—a pretty big deal on Wall Street. Because of the baby fat, I didn't have a single suit that fit. I searched and searched for a suit to fit my "unusual" shape. A colleague who knew a bit about being successful told me to have some suits custom made. How pretentious. Little old me, having suits custom made. Now I *really* felt like a big shot.

To be honest, I felt ridiculous, like a kid playing dress-up in grown-ups' clothes. Sounded like a practical solution to my problem, though. So someone at work told me about a company downtown that made his shirts for him. Wow, even his *shirts* were custom made! So they measured me, and I picked out a few designs. But the salesperson was new, and I didn't feel confident in her work. It probably would have been perfectly good for someone else, but God had a much bigger plan for me.

A few days later, I sat down with the Yellow Pages. Ah, the good old days before the Internet and Google and MSN directories. I was actually looking for a restaurant when the thought popped up that someone on Long Island might make suits. I saw an ad for Giorgenti, in Melville, Long Island. An Italian suit maker—I wasn't messing around! I love Italian clothes. I'd bought a pair of pants for my husband in Italy eight years earlier, and he was still wearing them, so I might have the same luck. Come to think of it, he's still wearing those pants today!

Janine Giorgenti met with me personally and was delightful. The first time I met her, she was eating what I believed to be the best breakfast on the planet: some pastries, a cup of coffee, and a bacon, egg, and cheese sandwich. The second time I met her, she was eating vegetables—for breakfast!

I almost ran out the door. Vegetables for *breakfast*? She must be nuts. Fruit for breakfast was stretching it, but Honey Nut Cheerios, flavored packaged oatmeal, chocolate Danish, or a bagel with cream cheese was really the only way to go. Right? Yeah, carbs, grease, sugar, and coffee—all the major food groups. That's what I called hardy.

When my friend Mitchell told me about his low-carb diet—he ate just an apple for breakfast—that was bad enough, but now this. Should I really trust someone this weird to make my suits, to be pinning me and nipping and tucking me? I mean, vegetables for breakfast? Wouldn't touch that one with a ten-foot pole.

Janine said she had gone to see this couple because she and her husband weren't feeling great. They had both wanted to do something about it. She was popping vitamins, too—more than I could imagine.

"Have you heard of alternative medicine?" she asked.

I thought, *Oh, please! That stuff doesn't work.* My diet consisted of pasta, pizza, candy, pastries, and any other kind of carb and dessert I could lay my hands on. Once in a while, I had a salad—Caesar with chicken, which I thought was on the extreme end of healthy. I did eat lots of fruit, though— apples, tangerines, or bananas that I bought just about every morning from Mohammed's fruit cart on the way to work.

So here I was, barely knowing this woman, and she was telling me I should eat vegetables for breakfast. I decided to let it go because she knew what she was talking about when it came to suits. We were at probably my fourth fitting when the truck hit. Cancer. When I couldn't make my next fitting, she said I should call those people—the vegetable people.

Oh, yeah. Not on your life.

"No, really. You should see what they have to say."

"Okay, I'll call them."

Well, I didn't call for several months, because I was a little tied up with the whole cancer thing. When I did, it was just as I'd suspected: Richard talked about things as if he were from another planet. He started explaining things to me about microscopes and pH balance and acidity, supplements and endobionts and other things I'd never heard before.

This was too far out there for me. I occasionally took a vitamin, and that was it. I later found out that some hard-encased multivitamins, such as Centrum, all end up undigested at the bottom of your cesspool. Yes, our cesspool guy confirmed that this had been his experience. So I thanked this very nice vegetables-for-breakfast man and went to chemotherapy.

My suits had been put on hold until after I finished the treatments. I loved Janine, even with that kooky little diet of hers. Well, after Kevin's diagnosis and my stage 4 diagnosis, I decided it was time to get the vegetable guy's number again. This time I actually made an appointment.

I prepared to enter the twilight zone. After all, I still had never been in a health food store. My diet did get a little bit better after the first bout of cancer. I didn't eat a whole container of Häagen-Dazs chocolate chocolate-chip, for example—I cut it down to half, with maybe only half a jumbo bag of M&M's every week. Believe it or not, I was still only a size 6 or 8, but I trusted my instincts. When you're guided toward something, no matter how crazy it might seem, take that step.

When my husband and I walked into Richard and Mary's office, I knew it would be a novel experience for me. You have to understand that we came from very different environments. We were two kids from Queens. I was the daughter of a police detective and worked on Wall Street. I'd had no exposure to alternative lifestyles. The place smelled of incense, and there were Chinese things scattered about and a spiritual bohemian theme. I thought it must mean they were flower children. Not that it was a bad thing, just an observation coming from a naive kid from Queens.

I shortly discovered that they were professional. It was calming, I have to admit that. Little did I know that I would soon be striving for a similar lifestyle. I learned that you can't judge a book by its cover. It turned out they were brilliant.

I saw a huge microscope with all kinds of equipment hooked up to it. Was this going to hurt? Richard pricked my finger with a lancet, then put a couple of drops of blood on several slides.

I was really surprised at how the blood looked under the microscope. I thought it would look like nice, round cells with a red background. It was anything but. Everything was smashed together, and it was full of black chunks.

"What's all that black stuff?" I asked.

"Open your mouth," he said.

Kind of an odd answer, but I figured, *What the heck, it's already weird enough.* So I opened and said "A-a-ah, just like a kid getting a physical.

He smiled. "You don't have to say 'a-a-ah.'"

Okay, I felt like a silly kid.

Very matter-of-factly, Richard said, "You have mercury poisoning."

Mercury poisoning? How could that be? I'd broken a thermometer as a kid trying to stay home from school one day—I lit a match under it until it exploded. Those little silver beads were really cool, especially when I rolled them around. But could that really have caused me to have poisoning?

"You have a lot of fillings," he said.

That was the understatement of the twenty-first century. Just about every tooth in my mouth had fillings on top of fillings on top of fillings (thankfully excluding the front teeth). You remember my healthy diet of pasta, pizza, and candy? Well, Mentos, Sour Patch Kids, Swedish Fish, and SweeTarts were among the top five—not exactly easy on the teeth.

Not only did I have a lot of fillings, but several years earlier I had gone to a new dentist, who recommended replacing the metal fillings with white composite ones. That sounded really good because the metal ones looked terrible. Unfortunately, the concept of composite fillings was relatively new, and those Mentos and SweeTarts ate them up. So, thinking the new dentist was a quack, I went back to the old dentist, who recommended putting metal fillings back in. So I did.

Needless to say, it seemed as though a lot of mercury from the fillings had been released into my body. When mercury fillings are drilled out or when you chew, mercury becomes like a vapor and goes into the brain, bloodstream, and other tissues. It is believed to affect the brain, heart, emotions, nervous and immune systems, and reproductive system among other things. If you've ever seen mercury in a dentist's office, the container has the skull and crossbones on it. Yup, it's a deadly poison.

It turned out that Richard was a freakin' genius. He told me all sorts of things about myself—stuff he couldn't possibly have known.

"Do you have chronic fatigue?" he asked.

"Yup."

"Do you have headaches?"

"Yup."

"Do you have sinus problems?"

"Yup, yup, yup." How could he possibly know?

"Do you eat a lot of sugar?"

He's scaring me.

"You don't eat a lot of vegetables, do you?"

Now it really felt like the twilight zone. This guy must have had a private detective on me. He was either a genius or psychic. I wasn't sure whether to stay or run, but I was fascinated enough to give him a few more minutes.

Kevin seemed completely unaffected. Have I mentioned that it's really hard to blow his mind? I don't think he's ever said anything was "amazing," yet that's one of my top five most-used words. He could see the most marvelous movie of all time and say, "Yeah, that was good."

Anyway, Richard made some notes and asked more questions. I got a little nervous. I thought he might get really personal and ask how often we had sex. He didn't. He was a real gentleman.

Within minutes, my perception had changed. My judgment had come from a place of fear. These two were truly brilliant and wonderfully kind. Mary had also had stage 4 cancer, and her lifestyle had been like mine. When she got her diagnosis, she changed her entire life and diet. In the eight years since then, she had lived cancer free. They must have known what they were talking about!

Kevin was up next. More of the same—questions Richard couldn't possibly have known, like "What happened in your head four or five years ago? Some kind of accident or surgery?"

Holy cow! He didn't have just any old private detective on our tails—he'd hired freakin' Columbo. The brain hemorrhage had happened four and a half years ago!

This was blow-your-mind kind of stuff. I had no idea how he knew those things, but he knew something. I definitely started to think there could be something to this—enough that if Richard said he thought they could help, I'd give it a try. He and Mary really seemed caring. If I didn't try it, I had only my life to lose. I would have climbed Mount Everest and stood on my head naked if that were what I needed to do to live.

Then came the million-dollar question, the one I had been sitting on the edge of my seat for hours wanting to ask: "Do you think you can help me?"

"It's very serious," they said, "and it needs to be dealt with as strongly as possible if you're going to survive, but yes, we think we can help you."

Richard said I still had a "barely decent constitution" (whatever that meant), so that would help. That was all I needed to hear. That was the climax of the whole day: "I think we can help you." Those words were joyous, spectacular, uplifting, amazing. Kevin, do you hear that? It's *amazing*!

I felt like Julie Andrews in the Austrian Alps, spinning around with my skirt billowing around me. I wanted to start singing, "The hills are alive with the sound of music." No one else had said they could help me.

"I'll do whatever you tell me," I said. Then I asked the *two*-million-dollar question: "Can you help Kevin?"

"Yes, we think we can help him, too. He's much stronger than you and will do well."

At that point, I cried—tears of joy, of course. Oh, what the heck, I hugged them!

Chapter Twelve

YES AND NO

Then came the tough part: the plan. Richard really did tell me to eat vegetables for breakfast. Not only that, he told me to eat them for breakfast, lunch, dinner, and snacks. No candy, cookies, pasta, or delectable desserts?

"Not the kind of desserts you're used to," he replied. "The best way to reverse the cancer is to clean your body of all the chemicals and unhealthy blood, then build yourself up again. That's the premise of biological medicine."

Biological medicine was basically bio-logic—literally, the logic of the body. The point was to get to the root cause of why something happened, remove that cause, then build the body back up so it could function the way it was meant to. When that happened, the body was stronger and the cancer couldn't survive.

Then came the really tough part: implementing the changes. It entailed a program of multiple supplements and drops to be taken at different points during the day, including suppositories (that's right, the kind you stick up your butt—that way, it goes right to the lower intestines and liver). There were also lots of green juices, wheatgrass (what the heck was wheatgrass?) and vegetables, vegetables, vegetables.

So the girl who never ate a vegetable pretty much had to live on them. How ironic. I didn't even know how to *make* a vegetable. All right, what was the big deal? I had to eat some vegetables. I could do that. How bad could it be?

The downer came when I found out how much work it would take. The music came to a record-scratching halt. Sorry, Julie.

"You really have to be diligent," Richard said. "But we've seen very good results for people who stick with it."

They had one case where a woman drank nothing but wheatgrass for thirty days. They showed us the before and after pictures of her blood, and it was remarkable. What the heck was wheatgrass? You want me to drink *grass*? Smoke it, maybe, but *drink* it? Far out, dude.

They said they couldn't tell us not to do conventional chemotherapy and radiation. We had to make that decision on our own, but it would make it more difficult for the program to work. It would be very hard to keep up with the destruction caused by the chemotherapy. However, it was much better to combine the two than not to do the program at all. It would also help maintain the immune system and keep me stronger during the process.

Richard and Mary were the only ones to say they thought they could help. No one else had said that. And that was all I needed to hear. I left having hope for the first time while still wondering if this was really possible.

As we left, I felt Kevin's energy. He was trying to be supportive, but he was also being told to get on this diet. He wasn't a big pasta, pizza, and dessert eater, although he did imbibe often enough. For him, it was meat and snacks and ice cream. He'd never been the kind of guy who really warmed to being told he had to do something.

He also didn't like change. Actually, he *hated* change. He and change were like oil and vinegar. (Oh, that's right, we couldn't have vinegar anymore, either. Thank goodness I could still have oil.).

Kevin didn't think what they were saying was possible. Was this a scam? A lot of yeast. Isn't that what you use to make bread? We didn't even know if they were making it up. They'd used words like "thrombocytes." Turns out a thrombocyte was a platelet crucial to normal clotting, but it sounded so mysterious.

Kevin thought it was all too far out there and that we'd wasted our money. After all, we were being treated at an excellent hospital. Why hadn't they told me about this? Kevin was one of the biggest skeptics. If it wasn't in his safe, familiar little box, he didn't want to know about it, and he would be the first one to admit it. I would have done anything to live. I didn't care what he or I believed or didn't believe—I was way too young to die.

I kept thinking about my beautiful, funny, adorable, affectionate, sweet little girl. I was also terrified of dying. Worse, I was terrified of dying of cancer. Worse than that, I was terrified of all the pain. The thought of the excruciating pain of dying of cancer was incentive enough.

So we left with what we could and couldn't eat, our new diet, our supplements, our instructions, our shopping list for more supplements to buy at the health food store (most of which I'd never heard of) and a tremendous amount of confusion and skepticism—and hope. That was the one gift beyond all gifts: hope.

The diet was basically broken down into two categories: yes and no. The "yes" foods were a whole lot of greens, some nuts, and a couple of grains (though I had to avoid the grains for the first month). The "no" foods were my entire diet. No pasta, pizza, candy, cookies, sugar (including honey), beans, vinegar, and more. No chicken parmigiana hero sandwiches, either.

Since I had no idea what to eat, I neglected to eat much. But I did drink quite a bit of wheatgrass—about eight ounces a day. Because the cancer was coming through the skin on my breast, I even put wheatgrass compresses on my skin. I bought juice from the health food store near my office and did my best.

There was no cookbook, no real instructions for a clueless health boob like me. I didn't even recognize most of the ingredients in the recipes I did find. So I called Richard and Mary regularly. They were overly patient and guided me like a little child going off to school for the first time: with love, compassion, and encouragement. So what the heck—I loaded up on wheatgrass, green juice, and green shakes. Anything green. Shrek would have fallen in love with me.

The first two weeks were hell. I was hardly eating, and going through a major detox. Did I mention that in the past I also drank eight cups of coffee a day, loaded with sugar—probably two to three teaspoons in each cup? So I was going through a heavy-metal detox, a coffee (caffeine) detox, and a sugar detox all at the same time.

And my body was reenacting the entire Civil War because I had dared feed it vegetables after all these years. I had a horrific, debilitating headache (and even that is an understatement), and I was sick to my stomach. I wanted to put my head down on my desk and go to sleep, but the thought of moving was unbearable. There was no way to relieve the misery.

And after work, I still had a three-year-old daughter who needed my attention. I had already taken time off for the surgeries and doctors' appointments, so I couldn't take more time off. My employer was very patient and understanding, given that I had been working there only a couple of months.

Richard and Mary also wanted me to see a dentist about having the mercury removed and having any root canals or infections treated. The dentist replaced three fillings on one side of my mouth and did something with a laser that prevented me from chewing for a week. I was miserable.

Giving up all the foods I loved really stunk. But you know what? I wanted to live. Was the type of food really that important compared to my life?

I couldn't watch TV, because every single commercial was an ad for food I couldn't have. I couldn't go into the supermarket, because all I saw was food I couldn't eat. I couldn't go out to eat. Plain and simple, the first two weeks sucked. Someone who wasn't as toxic and deteriorated, or someone who had at least had some vegetables in their diet, might not feel so bad.

By the end of the third week, things started to let up. The headaches were still there, but the nausea was subsiding. I got a little better at figuring out what to eat. By the end of the fourth week, I woke up, put my feet on the floor, and said, "I'm not tired." I had to think about it for a minute to see if it was true. Yup.

I let that sink in. For the first time in my life—in my *life*—I wasn't tired! I actually had never known what it was like not to be tired. Ever since I was a child, I had always been exhausted. I remember one time speaking to someone at work who wanted to know why I was always tired. I was shocked. "Aren't *you* always tired?" I asked. I had really thought everyone felt the same. Now that I think about it, she ate a lot of salads.

So when I put my feet on the side of the bed and realized what it was like not to be tired, I was dumbfounded. Then I could have jumped for joy and started to sing. Move over, Julie Andrews! This was what it was like not to be tired. The headaches and nausea were also gone. So were the sinus problems.

By the end of the fourth week, I had never felt better in my life. Oh, my God! I couldn't believe this was what I'd been missing. Yes, that's right: I had felt sick and tired all my life. Not one day had I felt great, all the way back to childhood.

I remember being at dance class when I was ten and having such horrific headaches, I needed to sit out. After four weeks, I begged my mother to let me quit. I remember being in school and not being able to concentrate or stay awake, so I zoned out and sat in the last row so the teacher couldn't see I was sleeping. When I went home, I tried to study to make up for what I'd missed in school.

I'd had chronic fatigue, chronic sinus problems, stomach problems, and chronic headaches. Several times every day I took Advil and Sinutab or Tylenol Sinus, and not one single doctor, in all those years, with all their tests, could tell me what was wrong. Can you imagine? And here I was after thirty-five years, feeling great. That was *amazing*. I wanted to call Richard and Mary and tell them how much I loved them!

Ultimately, Richard and Mary put me on the path that saved my life. The medical tool that saved my life was the microscope. Isn't it ironic? The one thing I had doubted most had saved my life. The people we had been the most skeptical about saved my life. The ones we had trusted most, the doctors, couldn't help and had misdiagnosed me.

If I had listened to the doctors, I wouldn't be here today. That couple turned out to be the sweetest, most caring and loving, most special people. They put me on a path and guided me along the way. My family and friends also supported me devotedly, no matter how bizarre things seemed. Without that support, I wouldn't have been able to stay on the path.

A month after our first appointment, it was time for my follow-up appointment with Richard and Mary. I was in a bit of a panic. This was the deciding moment. If it hadn't worked at all, I was screwed. They were my only hope. The big question was, "Is there hope?" I had done the best I possibly could, and faced the last gunfight at the OK Corral. Even so, it still could be *hasta la vista, baby.*

I would like to say Kevin did as well with the diet, but he was truly miserable. It required so much change, which was tough for him. He hated being told what to do. He was angry about his cancer, and he was even angrier about mine, which was understandable. At times, he was like that angry lady in the doctor's office, ready to jump across the room and rip someone's head off. Other times, he was perfectly fine. But this part, the changing-diet part, made it all a little too real.

I had no patience. I wanted to know. The same ritual ensued: the finger prick, the slides, the monitor. I was more than a little surprised. The blood looked very different this time. There were actually some round cells. I turned to Richard and asked, "Where's all the black stuff?" About 90 percent of it was gone. Gone.

"You've cleaned it out," he said.

I was in shock—jaw-dropping, speechless shock. There must have been a magic trick somewhere. I wondered if he'd changed the slides. Were the images prerecorded? All those questions that a naive, negative, mistrustful, fearful novice would think. But I had watched him like a hawk. I'm a suspicious detective's daughter, after all. I even looked directly through the microscope to make sure the slide went with the picture. They were exactly the same. There was no trickery, no smoke and mirrors, only honest-to-goodness science.

"How are you feeling?" he asked.

"I feel better than I've ever felt in my life."

He smiled. "That's very good."

In that moment, I knew he really wanted this for me. He explained that I felt better because my blood was so much better. There was a direct correlation between the blood and how someone felt, and the blood didn't lie. When the blood was sick, the person felt sick. When the blood was healthy, the person felt healthy.

This must be someone else's blood, I thought, smiling to myself. Yet I felt the excitement of a kid at Christmas, wondering if that really was her bicycle under the tree. So I asked the million-dollar, knot-in-the-stomach question: "So, do you think you can *still* help me?"

"Oh, yes," Richard said. "I do think you can be helped. But it's actually you who will be helping yourself. In fact, after seeing how well you've done, I'm very optimistic. If you continue to do what you're doing, I believe you'll be able to reverse the cancer."

YES! I punched the air with my fists, like a runner who has just crossed the finish line first. I wanted to kiss him.

I couldn't wait to see Kevin's blood. I was still terrified about his cancer, and he hadn't been able to keep as strictly to the diet. The finger prick, the slides, and the monitor. Well, his blood looked pretty good, too. I was happy for him—and a little ticked. How had he been able to get such good results doing only 70 to 80 percent of the program while I worked my butt off for 100 percent?

"You see," Richard said, "the weaker your constitution, the harder you have to work. All those years of being sick and taking over-the-counter medicines, having chemotherapy, the mercury poisoning, eating a terrible diet, having some really horrible traumas, a really tough childhood, and food allergies broke down your constitution."

Kevin, on the other hand, hardly took any type of medicine, felt relatively good (until he had a little brain hemorrhage and some cancer, that is), hadn't eaten nearly as much pasta, pizza, and candy as I had, had never had metal fillings, and hadn't had chemotherapy. He had taken interferon and a vaccine, which had aimed to strengthen, not break down, the immune system. There's got to be something to that. So his drop of blood looked nice and round and red and full. He felt better, too.

Wow! I left there feeling excited. Now I had real evidence to back up the belief that they could help me. That defining moment of seeing the improvement in my blood changed the whole course of my life for the better. Now my scientific, logical mind received the confirmation my heart had been hoping for. If I had not seen the improvement in my blood with my own eyes, correlated directly to the way I felt, I would not have continued on this path. Now there was something truly measurable to keep me on the path. I was a believer.

The elation lasted about ten seconds before the fear set in again. I was still terrified because I knew I didn't have much time to make this work. It takes two years of constant work to get mercury out of the body, and I didn't have two years. Even though the mercury had dramatically lessened, my body was most likely still loaded with it.

I had put off the decision long enough. Would I stick only with what Richard and Mary told me to do, or would I also do chemo? Richard never told me *not* to do chemo. He told me I had to make that decision. How could I possibly make that decision? What the heck did I know about alternative medicine?

I spoke to everyone looking for any shred of advice or information that would help me make a decision that might determine whether I lived or died. Now, I wasn't big on making decisions. Never have been. I prolonged them as long as possible, looking at every angle, making sure I had covered all the bases. This was a live-or-die decision. It was a total leap of faith to do what Richard and Mary told me—after all, it wasn't "standard protocol."

Silly me. I had no idea how lifesaving it was.

I ultimately decided to do both. I cut my ties with the hospital where Dr. Coldheart worked, and went to the hospital where my husband was being treated. Surprisingly, his oncologist did both melanoma and breast cancer. Hey, maybe we could negotiate a package deal—buy one chemo, get one free. Buy two chemos and throw in radiation.

We really liked the oncologist and trusted her. Unlike Dr. Coldheart, she wanted to do some kind of treatment. She had not written me off. She wanted to do whatever she could to help me. In fact, I overheard her talking to the radiation oncologist, who thought the treatment wouldn't work and was too risky.

"She's only thirty-three," the oncologist said. "Her husband has cancer, and they have a little baby. We have to do *something*."

So I felt great physically. Then I began radiation and targeted therapy. That was the end of the happy, feel-good trips to Richard. In fact, that was the end of my body having happy feel-goods. I started to feel like my old self again. The chronic fatigue, headaches, sinus problems, diarrhea followed by constipation, and hair loss returned. I cut my hair short again. I lost about half of it this time.

My blood started to look worse. I thought, *Well, this really sucks.* It's one thing to feel lousy and then feel lousier. It's another thing to feel great, even wonderful, and to have that taken away. That really sucked.

My oncologist encouraged me to go to the hospital support groups for advanced cancer patients. It wasn't for me. I needed to focus on the positive.

I know that support groups have helped millions. They can give you a sense of not being alone and show you that you're not the only one dealing with something. They can also be a great resource for information and services. But they brought me down.

I needed to focus on positive things. I wanted to share what I'd learned about the diet. Surprisingly, no one in the group wanted to hear about it. They spent the whole time in misery. I couldn't do that. I needed to take action in a positive way. Maybe a cancer inspiration group would have worked better.

The oncologist and the radiation oncologist were astonished at how well I handled the chemo and radiation. I was certain that it was due to the diet and supplement program. Even with all the side effects, I fared better than any other patient they had seen, especially given the type of treatment I was undergoing. One of the most impressive things was that my skin didn't burn from the radiation until the last couple of days. Considering that the radiation was hyperstimulated by the targeted therapy and lasted eight weeks instead of the traditional six, and that I kept forgetting to use the lotion, they were astounded.

They also didn't tell me not to take my supplements. They didn't want to know about it, but they also didn't pressure me to give them up. "Stage four is stage four," was their attitude. "There's not much we can do for you, so do whatever you feel you have to do." For that, I am eternally grateful.

Chapter Thirteen

THE CLOUDS ARE STARTING
TO BREAK UP: SWITZERLAND

We began the next phase of our journey roughly three months after I met Richard and Mary. Our destination was the Paracelsus Clinic. Not our usual vacation spot, but we hoped we would be able to look back thirty years later, knowing it helped us live those thirty years.

Our journey took us into the world of European biological medicine. Of all the alternative therapy clinics in the world, why did we choose the Paracelsus Clinic? That's simple. Richard had studied with Dr. Rau, the clinic's chief medical director. Dr. Rau received his medical education at Berne University in Switzerland, but he also passed the final American medical exams. His clinic was the first of its kind, even in Switzerland, and was highly regarded as a center for natural medicine.

Biological medicine actually made such logical sense, it's sad that it hadn't spread like wildfire throughout the States. Switzerland had already figured out how to remain at peace with the world; peace was crucial to the world's health equation and to our personal health equation. They had figured out how to make the best watches and the best army knives (though why a peaceful nation needs army knives, I don't know). It also made sense that they had figured out the logic of the body.

Let's look at the definition of "biological." "Bio" means "organic or life process"; "logic" means "sense," actually "common sense." Put the two together, and you have the logic, or common sense, of the body: "bio-logical."

It searches for the logic, or root cause, of the issue or illness, removes the cause, and supports the body so that it can strengthen and build itself back up to heal. This approach contrasts with treating only the symptoms of illness, which is the standard method of conventional Western medicine. Unlike the way chemotherapy is prescribed for cancer patients, there is no cookie-cutter treatment for everyone with the same disease. Instead, biological medicine searches for all the many factors that contribute to the illness, and addresses all the issues. In biological medicine, rather than use treatments that seem worse than the disease itself, practitioners strive for a treatment that boosts the body's own ability to heal. Amazing, right? Simple, right?

Nearly as simple as how I ended up in Switzerland. This is why I believe that when you raise your arms up in surrender and allow your eyes and your heart to gaze up to the heavens, and say to God or whomever you believe in, with all the trust, faith, and pleading you can muster, "God, just please show me the way," things start to happen. When you are ready to surrender your own ideas and be directed by a higher power, the guidance generally comes. Sometimes the clues are subtle, and you need to be on the lookout for unexpected synchronicities to show you the way. You just have to be willing to trust in—and act on—what shows up.

Take, for example, the way we wound up in Switzerland. During our first appointment with Richard and Mary, Mary turned to Richard and said with the quick-talking excitement of a native New Yorker, "I think they should go to Switzerland." She said it as easily as if she were saying, "I think they should go to the corner store and get a quart of milk."

Silence. Kevin and I nearly cracked our necks to see Richard's reaction. We waited while he contemplated the trip for a long moment. He pursed his lips pensively, then nodded. "Yes, I think that is a good idea."

Switzerland? Are you kidding me? As in across the Atlantic and half of Europe Switzerland, the Alps Switzerland, the land of milkmaids, yodeling, and cheese with holes in it Switzerland? First they want us to eat vegetables for breakfast; now they want us to fly halfway around the world, too. It got crazier by the minute.

"What exactly does that mean?" I asked. "Going to Switzerland?"

"There's a clinic where they have extremely effective treatments that aren't available here in the States," Mary said. "I think it will help jump-start your healing." Mary flipped through a Rolodex, scribbled something on a piece of paper, and handed it to me. "Here's a number to call. See if they can get you in right away. You'll probably have to go for three weeks."

"Thanks" was all I could muster amid the shock.

My family already thought I was crazy as a loon to be eating so many vegetables, salads, and green drinks, giving up my favorite Italian foods, and believing that diet and supplements would save my life. How were they going to react when I told them two people I had just met wanted me to go to Switzerland? And how about that job I had finally gotten after being out of work for so long? How would my boss feel about my heading off to the Alps? In the past, my concern for what others thought would likely have stopped me. But this time I was faced with a life-and-death decision. When someone seemed so certain and radiated the confidence Richard and Mary possessed, that little voice inside my head said very softly, *I think maybe we should go.*

I knew that self-interest wasn't behind their recommendation. They had nothing to gain by sending me to Switzerland—nothing but the satisfaction of helping someone who was sick and needed a new and alternative way to become well again. I knew at my core that they wanted to help us, that they wanted us to live. I later learned that Mary had broken down and cried after our first visit. She saw two young people with cancer and a little girl and didn't think that we would be able to accomplish all that we must to survive.

I wanted to live. Of that I was certain. And no one else had been so certain as Richard and Mary about what I should be doing to make that happen.

Here was the first step of healing: saying, "I will do whatever it takes to live." It meant that much to me. So Switzerland it was. Wasn't that right next to Austria? Maybe I could pop in on Julie Andrews and the Von Trapp family and we could do our rendition of "The Hills are Alive" together.

I wondered how I was going to pull that one off. I had only just started to earn a paycheck again. Our savings were gone. Was I nuts? How could I possibly do this? The little voice said, *Trust, Joyce, just trust.* It was speaking very softly but insistently.

One thing was sure: I wasn't going to let money keep me from saving my life or Kevin's life. What good would it be to stay out of debt but fail to save my life? How would my daughter feel? *Sorry, baby. Mommy decided it was more important that you have this extra money than have me to spend the rest of your life with.*

Well, that would have been silly. After all, I'd have a lot more earning power if I lived. I said to myself, *Self, if you need to do this, the money will come.* I thought that at the moment, and now, looking back, I'm certain. You believe it, you know it, you feel it, you trust it, and you expect it. That's how. Once again, if you just put your arms up and ask for help, it will come.

By the time I left Richard and Mary, going to Switzerland and pursuing biological medicine seemed like the most logical thing to do. I took the first step and contacted the Paracelsus Clinic in Lustmühle, Switzerland. They had a waiting list three months long. "I don't know if I have three months to waste," I said. "The situation is really bad and I need to get there right away."

A pleasant but serious Swiss German woman said, "Well, send us your medical records and a history. The doctor will take a look and we'll let you know what we can do."

So I filled out the form and sent that along with the records. They decided it was serious and that I should come quickly. However, most of their patients had cancer and had also been waiting, so they couldn't move it up much. I certainly didn't want to take someone else's place, so I vowed to work diligently with everything Richard recommended while I waited.

In the end, I had to wait until February, about ten weeks. Switzerland in February? Now, that would be interesting. We would fly into Zurich, then transfer to a train to St. Gallen. Someone would pick us up and take us to a small town named Teufen, to the Schützengarten, the inn where most patients stayed. If no one was available to pick us up, we could take another train to Teufen.

We had a few options on where to stay, but the Schützengarten made the most sense. It wasn't rated four stars, but it was clean and reasonably priced. We would be well cared for there. They cooked for guests and would follow Dr. Rau's recommended diet.

Mary kept saying, "You can go to Switzerland, but you can't eat their food. You have to stick to your diet."

You can go to the prom, but you can't kiss your date. You can go to the candy store, but only to window shop. You can go to the ice cream parlor but can't have any ice cream. Talk about tough. This was Switzerland, where they made the world's best chocolate! Ugh!

I asked Mary and the people at Paracelsus for the names of a few patients I could speak to before we left. That would make me more comfortable, and I might also get some tips. Mary had been to the clinic, but I wanted to get an idea of how other people had experienced it. The response was unanimously positive.

The only problems were the cost and Kevin's missing work. He wouldn't be able to stay all three weeks. Because I wasn't physically strong enough to make that kind of trip alone, my mother would come at the end and stay for a few days before accompanying me home.

We made all the arrangements and even got a really good deal on the airfare. We charged the whole trip, but our lives were first and money was secondary. Looking for something positive, we thought that at least we would have our tax refund after the credit card bills came in.

I believed the money would come. Some of it came before we even left for Switzerland. My brother Rich, five years older and always my protector, had looked out for me since I was a little girl. We grew up in a household of four kids. My two brothers were football players, and I was a swimmer. Even though we always had a meal on the table (which I had to guard with my life), there was little left for anything else. My mother stretched what income we had in creative ways. There were times when she rolled pennies to put enough gas in the station wagon so she could load us and our friends up and take us to the beach.

Rich was smart, had always been a hard worker, and found good after-school jobs. He looked for reasons to be overly generous, and when I was just twelve, he would give me fifteen dollars to wash his car or do a load of his laundry. Back then, fifteen bucks was a lot of money. He made sure I had some special things I never would have had otherwise. He gave me my first television—a twelve-inch black-and-white—and his air conditioner when he moved and it didn't fit into the window of his new pad. He stuck up for me if someone picked on me. For that, I will always be grateful. And once I got married, he looked out for Kevin, too. He brought him into the sometimes unstable power plant business and always made sure he had work. We always knew we could count on him, and we never had to ask.

We didn't turn to Rich for help when we planned to go to Switzerland— he came to us. That's just the way he was: very humble and the most generous person I know. Just as we prepared to leave for Switzerland, Rich handed me an envelope. He said it was from an anonymous collection taken up by people who cared about us and who wanted it to go toward our trip. The envelope was filled with cash. We were shocked, deeply touched, and humbled. To those who contributed, the gratitude that filled our hearts was overwhelming. Receiving that envelope gave us more than money; it gave us indescribable peace of mind.

*   *   *

So I packed our warmest clothes for our intercontinental trip. Traveling was much more difficult with the new diet, and we packed a cooler full of food. I grimaced as I passed all the shops in the airport. I was used to stocking up on candy for the plane rides, and I loved the Italian food on the planes. Sick, isn't it? I loved plane food—that's just crazy.

I was eating salads, young coconut, and livioli, a raw-food version of ravioli, which was actually really good, even for a pastaholic. What a relief it was to have my own food and not be tempted or have to panic about my next meal. We flew through the night and arrived a day later.

Making our way through the Zurich train station with my German language book and the help of some efficient signs, we loaded up the cart with luggage. I felt like Harry Potter on his way to Hogwarts as we got ourselves down through the terminal to platform nine and three-quarters. The train station made it feel like a magical, or at least mysterious, adventure about to begin. Getting to the platform required navigating passageways from the airport terminal, and even a ride on a frightening high-tech escalator that grabbed our luggage cart and kept it level while we descended to the platforms, and almost hurt ourselves trying to grab it back, like overprotective parents.

When we got to the train, a conductor was able to decipher my laughably poor attempts at German. He was fair-skinned, with an engineer's cap just like what one might expect on a Hogwarts train, and his handlebar mustache wiggled as he nodded vigorously and assured us that the train was heading to St. Gallen. "*Ja, ja,* St. Gallen." His nodding was contagious, so we nodded along with him, like three bobble-head dolls.

As we rode through the spectacular Swiss countryside, we were struck by the mountainous rural scenery that offered a sense of colorful lushness even in the dead of winter. The grass was a spectacular shade of glowing, almost neon green. The train cut through mountain passes, then emerged into sunlit rolling hills and farms dotted with grazing cows. Because we had flown through the night on a packed flight, Kevin and I tried to keep each other awake as we began to nod off. We missed the stop anyway.

When we got off two stops too late, we called the inn, and an adorable man named Christian arrived a short while later to greet us warmly. His excellent English was as comforting to us as a mother's soothing voice is to a newborn babe. He had a sweet smile, and we loved him right away. As we drove up the twisting, steep mountain roads, we learned that he had been an electrical engineer while his wife, Irene, worked in the Schützengarten.

Running the inn and caring for up to twenty patients at a time, shopping, cooking, and cleaning had become too much for her, and she needed help. As he explained, "I'd always worked with my head but had now wanted to work with my heart, Irene, so I joined her." Don't you just love when a man says something as sweet as that?

As the car climbed up the road, we caught our first glimpse of the Alps. Our breath caught as we took in the majestic view of the lush slopes and snowcapped peaks. It felt as if we were in a dream. Could we really be here, in Switzerland, witnessing one of God's most splendid creations?

The inn was just what I imagined a small Swiss inn to be. It was a creamy color outside, with brown wood trim. A few steps down to the left of the door revealed a garden tucked behind a fence, with a pretty little fountain in the center. I felt the excitement of a little kid finding a secret hideaway. At the inn, Christian's lovely wife, Irene, greeted us cheerily. We were at the point of dropping from exhaustion, but when we walked through the door, we immediately felt a sense of relief and safety. The inn was so cute, and Christian and Irene were cute, too, exactly as I had imagined. They regularly hugged, giggled, and smiled at each other. Just adorable.

The floors creaked as we entered through another low doorway with an old-fashioned latch handle. Our first glimpse inside revealed two small common rooms with two rows of tables that seated perhaps twenty people. Lace curtains framed all the windows. Sun filtered through and danced on the wooden floors. The ceilings were low, as they are in many old buildings in Europe. Making our way through the inn, we saw that the rooms were much smaller than what we are used to in the States—all a part of the Old World charm. One thing did stand apart from the otherwise thoroughly Swiss ambience: at the entryway, a Buddhist sand tray was available for guests to play with. To me, it brought a peaceful quality to the inn, adding to the feeling of being tucked in and sheltered.

Irene and Christian checked us in. She spoke excellent English and told us that the shuttle van would arrive shortly to take us to the clinic. We were introduced to Heinz, our driver, who had a lovely smile but spoke not a word of English to us beyond "Hello."

The clinic was a short ride away. We rode in silence, descending rapidly down the slick, winding road to the clinic, making one final stop at the hospital to pick up another patient. It was all very efficient (as I found the Swiss generally), and there was no time to give in to fatigue.

I was surprised to find that from the front, the building didn't appear large at all. Once inside, we realized it had been built very efficiently. Even the sliding glass entry doors operated with an efficiency and firmness that only the Swiss could create. The lobby was welcoming. A beautiful fish pond, glass elevator, and greenery made the small lobby feel welcoming. The staff was very kind and helpful, and I immediately felt at ease. When we arrived, the receptionist told us to wait for the American patient representative.

I was tired, but at least I was no longer as anxious. Most of the anxiety came from the anticipation of what the verdict would be. Would the doctors here agree with the hope Richard had given us? Had I been too naive, or was this trip to another continent the one thing that would bring us to the tipping point toward surviving? I felt that I was approaching the moment of truth.

After a brief wait, our American patient representative, Dalila, arrived. She sparkled with an energy and kindness that matched the environment. Her long, wavy dark-brown hair, olive skin, and dazzling smile matched her stylish clothing, and her help would prove invaluable. Her job, she explained, was newly created, and she brought abundant enthusiasm to her duties. She was neither European nor American but originally from Colombia. She answered all our questions and solved all our problems quickly yet in an unassuming, methodical manner, and we felt an ease and grace about her whenever she moved through the room. I quickly felt that I had made a friend. The trip had been very, very long, and we were quite tired, but she greeted us with such joy and enthusiasm, the fatigue became secondary.

Her name was pronounced "Da-lee-la," with a long "e," but I was only able to call her "Da-li-la," with a long "i," like in the radio talk show host's name. She didn't seem to mind. She sat down with us and explained in detail what to expect during our three-week stay, including a schedule that had already been planned out. Every minute was filled, including lunch breaks.

It took me back to fond memories of my high school days, when I would receive the class schedule for the year and feel the excitement and uncertainty of wondering who my teachers would be and whether my best friends would be in any of my classes. Now my schedule listed doctors and therapists rather than teachers. The only thing missing was study hall and gym. The course headings were also a little different: instead of chemistry and Spanish, it listed *darmbad, indiba, matrix regeneration therapie, zimmer,* and *ozon.*

The only thing that sounded even remotely familiar was *massage.* Did someone say massage? I'm beginning to like this place.

My first appointment with Dr. Rau was not at all what I expected. I found a tall, fit man with salt-and-pepper hair and an unassuming manner. He wore typical doctorly attire: white jacket, dark pants, black shoes, white shirt, and tie—all very professional. A goatee trimmed to his jawline added personality to his thin, kind face. He moved about the clinic with the excitement of a young boy, yet he had an aura of depth befitting a century-old sage. His compassion, warmth, and humility contrasted with my experience with many American doctors. His care and concern were etched in his eyes.

When asked a question, he appeared to listen not to the question but to what lay behind it—the root of the question. The search to find the root of a disease rather than merely treat the symptoms struck me during our initial conversation. After all, whenever a question is asked, isn't there usually something behind it? For example, "How effective are these treatments?" really means, "Am I going to die?"

Once the question was out, he contemplated for a few moments. He was obviously comfortable with silence. That was something new for this American used to immediate responses, even if they were inadequate. He sat silently and chewed on his pen cap, then answered very directly and thoughtfully. He was brilliant, down-to-earth, and understandable—no incomprehensible medical terms. I could listen to him talk for days at a time, and in fact, that is ultimately what I did. He was very serious yet kind, and he spoke excellent English.

The first part of the interview covered the specifics of my illness. Then he asked questions most doctors wouldn't normally ask: "What is really going on in your life?" "How is your marriage?" "Is your father living?" "What is your relationship with him?" "What is your dental history?" My relationship with my *father*? Wow. Was he kidding? What the heck does that have to do with the price of tea in China? Doctors back home examined you physically, then wrote you a prescription or two if you wanted. Baffled though I was, I found it all fascinating and sat on the edge of my seat waiting to ask the million-dollar question.

After each question, he stared at me long enough to make me feel awkward. He waited for answers, but he looked through me as if he could see straight into my soul. He chewed on his pen cap and eyed me pensively as if my answers didn't really matter—he was well past that. He was already figuring out what was really going on in my body and what blockages existed—something I would learn more about later. I got the distinct feeling that he knew me better than I knew myself.

I had to strip down. I glanced around the room to see who would hand me a gown. Nope, not happening.

Picking up on my confused expression, Dr. Rau chuckled and explained, "Americans are very prudish about their bodies. You get used to it very quickly here."

It seemed hard to believe that this serious, thoroughly professional doctor wasn't prudish about his body or anyone else's. While I had experienced my share of poking and prodding and lost most of my dignity during my thirty-six hours of labor and later with the mastectomy, I had always had that flimsy little piece of fabric that flapped in the breeze—I always had a gown. While I handled the immodesty better over time, I still wanted my gown, my blankie.

I gave in, and after stripping down to my underwear, I stood up as he held his hands about a foot away from my body, starting at my head and going down to my toes. He was getting an idea of my energetic strength. He said, "You have too much behind you here."

He moved his hand inward from about three feet away from my lower back, to about a foot away. "This is where you are living: in the past."

I was. He was right on from the moment we met. To my relief, he asked me to dress. I moved to another room, around the corner, where his assistant pricked my finger and put a few drops of blood on two slides, as Richard had done. Dr. Rau looked at my blood under the microscope, and it looked pretty bad to me. But he said he had a gut instinct I would be okay. After the way he had looked into my soul, I sort of believed him. That belief, or "faith," was the little bit of hope I needed to coax me further down this unusual path.

His next question was something of a riddle. "What would you do," he asked, "if it were five minutes to twelve?"

A Swiss expression, I gathered. "Um, what exactly does that mean?"

"It means it is five minutes before midnight, and midnight is the end of your life. You have only a short while to live. What would make you happiest?"

No one had ever asked me that before. In fact, I don't think I had ever asked *myself* that question. After a transcontinental flight, a few hours of sleep, a trip with Harry Potter, and all this newfound Swiss-ness, the question was rather deep. I was completely perplexed. I actually had no idea. I mean, I had a daughter. I would spend more time with her and my family and friends, but beyond that, no idea.

"Breast cancer patients put everyone before themselves, or they have a disappointment in a relationship with a partner or father," he explained.

He explained that another patient of his was in the same situation: stage 4, small children, although much heavier than I. When he had asked her the same question, she responded, "I should write a book. I have always wanted to write a book."

He told her to do it. When she said she didn't know how to write, they hired a ghostwriter for her. Soon she was touring on speaking engagements. That was five years ago.

"It is a great boost to the immune system to do something that makes you happy," Dr. Rau explained.

Well, I certainly had no intentions of writing a book or going on speaking engagements—that was crazy. I also didn't have any idea how to write—I'd never written anything but a term paper for school—but I got what he meant. Do something that makes you happy, whatever it might be.

I had no clue. Were we actually supposed to spend our lives doing things to make us happy instead of just work, work, work toward some goal or other? What about all the years of growing up and being told, *You have to work hard for whatever you want. Money doesn't grow on trees. Money doesn't come easily. Work, work, work. You can do more. You can do better.* Obviously, all with the best and most loving intentions for a better life. No mention of happiness ever entered into the equation in the Martin (my maiden name) household.

"Just think about the answer," Dr. Rau said. "Focus on being well and keep repeating, 'I am well.'"

He wanted me to spend some time with the psychologist. So I nodded, knowing full well that I was in no position to figure out what might make me happy. Instead, I got to work learning German and looked the words up in my phrase book: "*Es geht mir gut*" (pronounced "*ess gate meer goot*)—"I am well." Okay, but what makes me *happy*? That was too heavy to take on at the moment. Imagine that. Here I was, being asked to think about happiness, about joy, and it felt heavy and scary. Happiness—and thinking about it—should be light; it should lighten my mind and soul, shouldn't it?

Chapter Fourteen

THE LOCH NESS MONSTER

My appointment with Dr. Rau was followed by a lot of testing and evaluations. I underwent a dental exam and some dental tests. As a result of my sugar-filled history, even my *fillings* had fillings. At the clinic, I found out just how toxic the mercury was. During my stay, I learned a lot about dental work and about fixing the problems caused by the dental work—particularly the mercury amalgams—which played a big part in my recovery.

In addition to an extensive dental exam, they ran more tests. They did quite a lot of diagnostic testing to pull the whole picture together. "We don't treat the illness here at Paracelsus," Dr. Rau said. "We treat the *patient,* and every patient is different."

I was tested for food allergies. I found out that I was highly allergic to dairy, wheat, some nuts, eggs, and a number of other things.

Dr. Rau explained, "About three-quarters of the population is allergic to wheat and dairy, and they don't even know it. You are very allergic to them and must avoid eating these things. They are very harmful to you."

What's in just about everything we eat? You got it: dairy or wheat, or both. Not only do these things make those who are allergic feel lousy, but when we eat something we are allergic to, the immune system sees it as a foreign invader that it needs to attack. If the immune system is constantly working to attack food, then it doesn't have the strength to put its energy into fighting something like cancer. A strong immune system is our first defense in keeping our bodies strong and preventing cancer.

After this news, I started paying attention to what I ate and how it affected me. When I ate wheat, I started to get foggy and felt tired and more congested. When I ate dairy, I had sinus problems, head and chest congestion, and postnasal drip, and I coughed more. When I ate nuts, I had some of the same symptoms and a headache. There was my confirmation.

Kevin and I had separate schedules and appointments, so we passed each other in the halls and said hi. He was experiencing the same things from a very different angle—he was much more resistant than I. This "logical" type of medicine didn't blow his mind the way it blew mine. He was still fighting it. He felt it was enough that he was here. His attitude was, "I'm here. I'm doing it. That's all I can handle right now." I learned to focus on my own treatments, but I couldn't help wishing for his approval, his commitment. Still, the schedule allowed me to focus on my own experience and let go of his. The only time we had together during the day occurred at dinner, which we shared with other patients. We paid attention to our therapies and collapsed into bed each night.

As Dr. Rau requested, I waited for my first-ever appointment with the psychologist. Believe it or not, even with all I had been through, I had never been to a psychologist. But this wasn't your typical lie-on-the-couch-and-tell-me-about-your-childhood psychologist. This was a hands-on, let's-get-down-and-dirty-and-figure-out-what-makes-you-happy kind of psychologist. We identified many areas to focus on. Here are the main ones:

1. Focus on myself and what makes me happy. (At that point, I still had no clue.)

2. Focus on Kevin, Kelsey, and those who have been there for me.

3. Focus on the positives that came from the first bout with cancer.

Next, he gave me homework: to find the gifts that came out of my illness. This is what I wrote:

1. Getting closer to Kevin, even if it was occasionally extremely difficult.

2. Spending more time with my family.

3. The tremendous support, love, care, and concern that I received from friends and family.

Those were the things I should have been focusing on. I needed to focus on family and friends, rather than work. My family and friends had been there and given me so much when I needed it.

I realized I had been living in a very unhealthy, unbalanced way. I had put my efforts in the wrong place. I knew that and had for some time, but I had lots to work out. I needed to find out what would make me happy, what would bring me joy.

There it was again: a giant Loch Ness monster, rearing its ugly head to swallow me whole, while leaving alone all those people who knew what made them happy. Once I could come up with that, I then had to figure out how to build that into my life. That ought to be easy. Ha! Easy to say.

I continued with my homework by calling my best friend, Diane. She was watching Kelsey part of the time I was gone. I was immensely grateful, especially since she had two little ones of her own. How blessed I was to have a friend like her! She captured a room with her humor the moment she walked in, especially with her flowing blond hair and striking green eyes.

We had been born in Bayside, Queens, only six months apart, and lived next door to each other. So whenever I introduced her, it was not as "my friend Diane." I said, "This is Diane, my best friend since the day we were born." And she did the same. It was part of our title, our birthright, our badge of honor.

Then there were our parents, who had been best friends for over forty-four years, and our brothers, who were also best friends, and now our daughters were best friends. I called her parents Aunt Noreen and Uncle Jerry, and she called my parents Aunt Loretta and Uncle Dick. They were our cousins, maybe even closer. We had always been in each other's lives, even after they moved an hour away from us, when Diane and I were four.

Diane was the type of friend who knew what I was thinking before I had a chance to think it—who knew the answers before I had a chance to ask the questions. The type who knew exactly what to say before I even knew it needed to be said. The type who, patiently coming over after I slopped eight shades of the same color paint on the wall because I couldn't decide which one worked best, would chose one and say, "Oh, Joyce, why do you hurt yourself like this?"

When I was diagnosed the first time, Kevin and I had only recently moved into our home. There was quite a lot we had not yet accomplished, and we were just scraping by in more ways than one when I got sick. We had moved most of my parents' twenty-year-old furniture into our house and had pretty much just dropped the boxes wherever they fit. So we had chalky white paint on the walls and not a bit of anything new. A beautiful home, but definitely less than cheery.

Diane happened to be a talented interior decorator. So one day, as on so many days before my surgery, I was going through doctors' appointments and tests. That day happened to be one of the worst—the one with the callous plastic surgeon who showed me the baseball-stitched road map of my future chest and stomach, as if God had said, "Let me make her parts interchangeable, like Mr. Potato Head's." That was the day I threw up on the sidewalk.

It hit me the hardest that day because I realized this would not be "Let's get this over with so I can get back to work." This was the reality of lasting scars that would mark the devastation so I would never be able to forget. No matter how hard I tried, I would have a daily reminder every time I showered or put on my bra or bathing suit or got dressed or made love.

That day, I had arrived home to hear my friends, Diane and Dawn, calling me to my bedroom. When I opened the door, I was dumbstruck. My bedroom and master bath had been transformed. A new, colorful bedding ensemble was there, the furniture had been moved around, and coordinating decorative towels hung on a gold towel bar in the master bathroom. There were candelabras, a topiary potted plant, a dish of pearl bath beads on the platform tub fit for a Roman goddess, curtains, and a three-foot-high gold pedestal topped with an urn and a beautiful, flowing fern.

"I know you're going to have a tough recovery," Diane said with tears in her eyes, "and I wanted you to have someplace beautiful to be while you're feeling so lousy."

We all cried and hugged. They pulled this off in just a few hours. Talented, yes, but beyond that, her ability to see what I needed and just to do it before I even knew I needed it was awe-inspiring. I hadn't even thought of what recovery might be like. There are no words to describe what having a friend like that means, especially in the depths of a personal ordeal.

As a lifelong friend, she had certain privileges that others just didn't have, because no one else had earned them. She could lay it on the line and get a point across like an arrow nailing the bull's-eye, no matter how painful the truth was, and I still said, "Okay, thanks. I love you."

Part of the "happiness" homework quest was to ask someone who knew me well to answer the question "What are my strengths?" She answered as only my best friend since the day I was born could have: "You are such a moron," she said. "I can't believe you don't see them."

Uh, thank you? She then floored me with all the strengths that I didn't see in myself. She said, "You are the most generous human being walking the earth—not just financially but with your spirit and kindness—even to strangers. You are always there for people. You're reliable, dependable, intelligent, kind, loving, and kind of obsessive/compulsive, which has its pros and cons—it enabled you to survive, but it can make you and everyone else crazy, too. I know you will always be there for me. If I were in Ireland and told you I needed your help, you would be on the first flight out. Whatever you know, you want to share with everyone. You know that something better is out there, and you pursue it."

She brought me to tears. I knew that Diane loved me, but I could never have imagined all that she saw in me. I couldn't help but think she was biased. I did acknowledge that I might not always say or do the right thing, but my heart is always in the right place. When I recovered from my tears, I asked about my weaknesses. That was easy.

"Your weakness is this Martin family work, work, work mentality. It's ridiculous. You don't have enough time with Kelsey, because of your work. It's killing you, and it's breaking my heart."

"You're right," I said.

Both of us knew full well that I didn't have a clue about any other way to live. She was thrilled to hear I would be making changes. She was right: I was a moron. I hung up saying, "Okay, thanks. I love you. Call you tomorrow."

My second appointment with the psychologist didn't go as well as I had hoped. He was happy to hear that I now knew some of my strengths. But I was still stuck on figuring out what I wanted and what my fears were about having what I wanted. It all boiled down to low self-esteem, fear of what people thought of me, and not wanting to be selfish. The gist of the meeting was that to get better, I had to focus on myself. I had no clue how to do that, either. It just wasn't in my matrix.

The clinic did many different kinds of treatments, most of which would seem unusual to someone who had no experience with anything like them— that is, to someone like me. One was ozone therapy, which was done in some places in the United States. They hooked me up to an IV and took out some blood, mixed it with oxygen and some vitamins and homeopathic remedies, then put it back in.

It's supposed to give the patient energy. I didn't feel much better, but it did make me feel nauseated and gave me a metallic taste in the back of my throat. At another point, I also had a detox infusion. I didn't like it—it reminded me too much of getting chemo.

The hyperthermia treatment made me stink. No, really, I reeked like something out of a garbage Dumpster. They didn't want us to shower until the next morning, so I continued to stink everyone out of the room, the clinic, and the Schützengarten. Kevin didn't desert me, but I can tell you that no one else volunteered to sit with me at dinner. To really understand how bad I smelled, you must understand what hyperthermia is.

Whole-body hyperthermia was probably the single most effective noninvasive treatment that could be done in a four-hour period. Sadly, it was not available in the United States, which just showed the sorry state of affairs in our health system. It might sound awful, but the benefits blew away any discomfort. The purpose was to safely bring the body temperature as high as possible, up to 104 degrees.

The idea was that most people with cancer don't have fevers, because the immune system is unbalanced. The immune system is the tool our bodies use to self-regulate and fight cancer. Cancer hates heat, so the higher the heat, the more cancer it kills off. It was an amazing way to detoxify. Therefore, the reason I smelled so bad was because toxins were coming out of my pores.

This treatment was done with direct one-on-one monitoring. It happened in a room used only for that purpose. You strip down to a gown—the one time gowns are allowed. Everything else was au naturel—the European way, baby. Next, the patient is zipped into a soft box that encases the body. There is room to move around and plenty of oxygen. You can keep your head out, but putting it in is much better because that typically allows the body temperature to climb higher.

A personal nurse never left the room during the therapy. She provided infusions, monitored the patient (me), answered questions, provided water and cold compresses, played my favorite CDs, and even gave me a nice, cooling foot massage when things got really hot. The doctors also came in to check on me.

Dr. Rau preferred that patients not talk to anyone or do anything during the treatment, in the hope that the treatment might bring on an emotional experience, a breakthrough. Maybe something from childhood would come up and I would release it. Some people have great experiences. Nope, not me. It was just another job. Quieting my mind didn't fit into my equation. They gave me tips, like focusing on my breath: in through the nose, out through the mouth. When I tried to do that, I kept making a sound like a Bronx cheer, or "raspberry." It made me recall videotaping Kelsey as we blew noisily against her little belly when she was just a few months old and she did it back to us, laughing with glee.

I couldn't keep from laughing as I tried the breathing meditation. It reminded me of one night when Kevin and I had stayed at my brother Rich's house. Rich fell asleep on the couch after a party. He whistled as he breathed in, then made the raspberrylike sound as he breathed out, all the while wearing a silly grin—the funniest snore we had ever witnessed. Kevin, my sister-in-law Barbara, and I sat and watched him for over an hour, laughing so hard we could barely breathe. Laughter! I stopped myself. This was serious work for me.

I needed distractions, so I prayed and read a novel. Reading was a big no-no. Dr. Rau was not happy with me about that one—I was not being a very good student. I put Kelsey's picture above the glass opening so I could look up at her while she looked down at me. She was my inspiration for getting better.

It was an adorable picture of her in her red satin and velvet dress from Christmas. I wanted to squeeze those perfect, precious cheeks. I kept thinking about the hug I would get, and all the missed kisses, when I arrived at the airport back home. Whenever Kelsey hadn't seen me for a while, she dropped everything and ran at me screaming, "Mommy-y-y-y-y-y-y-y!" in one long, continuous exhalation. She really tried to knock me down, and sometimes she did. Then we laughed hysterically as people at the airport stepped over and around us.

I meditated and visualized that the infusions were bringing all these great little bouncy stick figures into my body. They were building up my immune system. I visualized the white cells dancing while happily eating up the black stuff. I also had a fish swimming all through my body, eating the cancer as if it were fish food. As it swam, Kelsey was holding on to its tail and squealing with laughter.

I imagined the infusion flowing through my body and washing out the cancer and giving me clean, healthy blood. The white cells were dancing to the CD the nurse played for me: Belafonte singing, "Day-o, da-a-ay-o, daylight come and me wan' go home." Don't you know that when my blood went under the microscope again, it had lots of those bouncy stick figures in it! I was beginning to believe that visualization really did work. You might say, "Of course it works, silly—it's been proven for centuries." What did I know?

Hyperthermia was done once a week if the patient was strong enough. At one point, on a shorter trip when I was a little stronger, I did two in one week, five days apart. My temperature usually ranged from 103 to 104. I was ecstatic when I reached 104, though I was able to reach that on only two occasions before I bailed out.

I know 104 sounds crazy, but it's not nearly as uncomfortable as when you have the flu—mainly because you don't have the other symptoms, like vomiting or stuffy head or body aches. The main side effect was that I was hot—really, really hot. I got a headache and was dizzy afterward, which made sense. Don't get me wrong—I was praying for it to be over. But still, when it was over, I actually looked forward to the next hyperthermia treatment. No, not because I'm masochistic, but because the benefits were so powerful.

Some of the treatments seemed pretty bizarre until I was brave enough to ask what they were. Matrix regeneration therapy, or MRT, for instance. For this treatment, the end of a hose attached to a huge vacuum pump was pulled from my spine to my sides in one-inch intervals. It suctioned out toxins. Weird, but hey, I was game.

Next they used little rolling metal balls that connected an electrical stream to a metal plate that I lay facedown on. They rolled the balls across my back. In his best English, the therapist explained that the polarity of the cells in the body was something like a field of corn. Some cells were standing up and some were lying down. The MRT affected the polarity and made them all stand up like soldiers. After playing roller ball, I got a shoulder massage. Now we were talkin'!

I really enjoyed sitting out on the balcony of our little apartment at the inn. I loved it there. One glorious part of being there was that I really had so little other than myself to worry about—just my next appointment, juicing, making the bed, and my next meal. It was such a nice reprieve from the real world.

Guess what? They roughly prepared the Paracelsus diet, which was cooked, not raw, at the inn. Food had become a bit of a dictator. Irene was an awesome cook, and wasn't it great that I didn't have to fix it myself! I would walk in the door and ask, "What's for dinner?" I probably made her crazy, but I couldn't help myself.

Very little was raw—quite liberal compared to our diet. I ate lots of salads, and she loaned me a juicer I could keep in the apartment. We had a kitchen in our room, and Kevin juiced for me every morning. It was going to be tough when he left.

I walked up to the grocery store and bought a few things to juice and some peppers to snack on. Fresh organic produce was rare and expensive, but there were staples like celery, English cucumbers, and spinach. I juiced every day, happy to avoid the awkwardness of asking Irene to make it. She was about the busiest, most efficient person I knew, and she certainly didn't need one more thing to do.

Since the clinic was closed on weekends, we took those days off. Then, after the first week, Kevin left to give Kelsey a big hug and kiss for me. The sun was shining as I sat on the balcony, sipping a tasty cup of detox tea. It was like springtime. The birds chirped as I gazed out at the most spectacular view of snow-covered mountains that seemed so close, I could have reached out and scooped up the snow. Then I'd wing a snowball at that gi-normous bell swinging from Elsie the cow's neck, just for kicks, just to hear it ring.

Listening to the birds in a little piece of paradise, I felt at peace for those few moments—something I don't think I had truly experienced before. The church bells were ringing. I sipped my tea and drank it all in. I thought for a moment what it would be like to live like this. It was so much simpler than the life I had created at home.

Chapter Fifteen

My Mom: My Rock

Mom arrived at the end of the second week to take over support at the clinic and to escort me home again. She was such a cutie. She just loved this stuff. Any new experience made her so excited. I definitely knew where I got that from!

She had handled all our trials remarkably well—at least on the outside, for show. You can imagine the anguish and pain she experienced watching my husband, my daughter, and me endure all this. She had always been an angel, sent to whoever needed her.

Sadly, taking care of people took over much of her life. Immediately after she had married, her mother had a massive stroke that left her paralyzed and mute. Mom moved in with my nana and cared for her from that time until Nana's death fifteen years later. She raised four children practically by herself and worked while my father worked three jobs to put us through Catholic grammar school. They lived hand to mouth without an extra penny for anything, yet she always still managed to find a way for us to have fun.

Imagine watching your child, your baby (every mother thinks of her child as her baby even if that baby is seventy), go through all our ordeals. To stand by your child as her husband is paralyzed and has brain surgery, to watch her baby go through the gut-wrenching decision of whether to abort, to watch that same daughter go through the agony and fear of cancer, then to watch her daughter's husband go through the same.

On top of the physical ailments, add financial ills. She had watched her daughter lose her job. Then she had been told that same daughter was going to die. All this by the time her child was thirty-five, and all within a five-year period. How much could one mother bear? I think it may have been worse for my mom than for me.

Finally, after rushing back from Florida each time she got the devastating phone calls, when Kevin was diagnosed with cancer she figured, okay, enough was enough. She and my father sold their home in sunny Florida. It had been modest, but it had been her retirement. She gave up her dream and moved back to Long Island permanently. She moved into a two-bedroom apartment to care for us and our infant daughter again and again, living day to day with the worry.

Every mother's worst anguish is to witness her child's suffering. No mother should ever have to watch her child suffer. Mom cooked, cleaned, shopped, did laundry, changed diapers, fed our baby, and ran our household. She drove me wherever I needed to go when I couldn't drive myself or when I needed the emotional support. Her physical endurance should have earned her a gold medal.

When I found an alternative method to fight the cancer, she took care of Kevin and Kelsey while I was out of the country. She even flew to Switzerland. She juiced vegetables for me and learned a whole new way of thinking and preparing raw foods for our healing. In short, she paved the road to recovery for me with her blood, sweat, and tears. And she did every bit of it with such love.

She is my pillar of strength, truly a guardian angel God had blessed me with, knowing I would need her to endure the challenges. There was no way to give back to her all she had given. I can only hope that whatever I give her now will be joyful times filled with fun, rather than the dread of that next phone call.

How can I express my gratitude for God having given me this mother? She is such a joy to be around. She is probably the most giving person I've ever met. I really lucked out. She sacrificed so much for us and worked so hard to help us heal. It was never, "Well, maybe you can get better." It was always, "You *will* get better," no matter how much she was dying inside. I was worth so much to her, she devoted her life to helping me live.

God was so good and shed blessing after blessing on us. My illness and my mother have been among my greatest blessings.

Mom arrived on Sunday when everything was closed, which was pretty cool. It reminded me of when I was a kid and everything closed on Sunday and we always had family dinner together. Now nothing is closed, ever.

We went to church that morning. It was in German, of course. My mind was all over the place. It was very hard to say the Apostles' Creed in English while everyone else said it in German. The words went right out of my head. I also tried saying the rosary. I had no clue what else was going on, so what the heck. Couldn't do that, either.

They had a men's choir, which sounded lovely. The funny thing was, they sang a song in English. "I vant to go to heaven vhen I die, I vant to go to heaven vhen I die, I vant to go to heaven vhen I die. Oh, Lord, vhen I die."

It was a combination of singing and yodeling, which was just the cutest and most beautiful thing, but I also couldn't help chuckling. The people were so happy there, not uptight or in a big rush. They had a lightness to them. They laughed a lot. The people at the clinic laughed a lot, too. They loved what they did, and loved working at Paracelsus. Sure, there was stress and pressure, but they handled it so beautifully, much better than I feel we do in the states. They seemed to have more balance. I wanted to move there!

The nurses had voices like angels. No kidding. There was a certain beauty about the way they spoke, especially given the firm precision of the German language. They had a singsong way of speaking that sounded so happy, it made me feel better just listening to them. They were so helpful, too. If I needed this or that, they were very patient. Also, meeting the other patients was great. It was comforting to feel immediately at ease because I wasn't the only sick person. Instant camaraderie. It was like an inspirational support group. I learned just as much from them as I did from the treatments.

It really was the environment. The energy and the people made it a healing experience unlike any other. Its cleanliness was pristine. Rooms were often bright and sunny, although it could be a little gloomy in winter due to the rain and snow and shorter days. One of the things I liked most was that it was a much healthier way of being sick and of healing than in the States, and there was so much more hope that patients would get better.

I saw many of the other patients and staff throughout the day. It was nice to say hi to a familiar face while thousands of miles from home, even if I had known the person only five minutes. Patients had meals together, as well. It was nice to walk into the restaurant at the inn or the clinic and feel comfortable sitting with someone I didn't know.

That had always been very difficult for me. I felt pretty anxious when I didn't know anyone and needed to get in there and start a conversation. It's hard to believe, but I was actually really shy and self-conscious in new situations. Here it was different. It was still hard, yet easier than other times because we already had something in common.

Within minutes we had a synopsis of each other's medical history. Some patients were from America; others were from various places all over the world. Sometimes language was a barrier, but we usually had at least one person who could translate. When patients spoke the same language, they often sat together anyway. When people heard Kevin and my story, they kept saying, "You should write a book."

"Oh, no, no!" I chuckled. "Not me. I'm no writer."

I made a friend from the States, named Sandra. We both had stage 4 cancer. Sadly, sometimes our illness becomes our identity. *You know her, the one with stage 4; he's the one with MS; he's the one with prostate cancer.* It wasn't meant in a bad or limiting way; it just was how it naturally happened, I guess. She was doing a diet similar to mine—having a hard time but doing well. It was harder to stick to it at Paracelsus because they had very little raw food. Most things were cooked, and they didn't have juicing, though they did have salads.

We spoke with a lovely older woman. She was eighty-three and had been given six months to live after being diagnosed with colon cancer. She had come to the clinic then. Six years later, she was still here. She had been on the Rau (not raw) diet. She spoke a few languages, had traveled around the world while working for the Red Cross, and lived in Switzerland. I loved meeting so many interesting people and hearing all the inspirational healing stories.

Johan was a patient very sick from heavy metal toxicity. He had chronic headaches and pains in his teeth and jaw if he got too close to a television. No doctors could figure out what was wrong—until he arrived at Paracelsus.

Before going there for treatments, he couldn't work in front of the computer for more than fifteen minutes without severe pain. By the time we met, he was able to work up to an hour. He gave me a pyramid to put on my head to help with the headaches caused by the heavy metal detoxing. Sounded crazy, but hey, who was I to argue?

It worked. It was a metal frame in the shape of a pyramid, about eight inches wide and eight inches high. It was made of gold. I wore it for only a few minutes, but three hours later I really did feel better. If you put an apple under the pyramid and another next to it on the counter, the one under the pyramid would still be fresh after the one outside the pyramid had rotted.

The Egyptians built them to preserve bodies. It worked for all those centuries. It had something to do with the energetic construction. Irene told me about a clinic in Germany where the beds sat at a very specific point midway through two connected pyramids. They put people with cancer in there and they were cured. Again, who was I to argue?

As I was learning, there is much outside mainstream medicine that works. But why was it such a secret? It was empowering to feel that I was taking responsibility for my health. I actually felt as if I was already healthier just by doing something toward improving my health. Okay, so the treatments weren't always that much fun. Most were actually fine—a time to chill out, take a break from the real world. Not much else to worry about, other than making it to the restaurant before lunch was over. *I wonder what Irene is making today?*

*   *   *

After about two weeks, I came up with a list of things I loved. Yes, it took the full two weeks. The list wasn't earth-shattering, but hey, it was a start! I realized I enjoyed watching old movies, springtime, breathing in the air on a sunny day, watching the pink, purple, and yellow crocuses push up out of the ground, traveling to historic places and seeing the way other people lived. Caribbean beaches, of course, and the excitement of a snowstorm and being shut in and watching it through the window, hoping for a foot at least. A nice fire, watching Kevin and Kelsey play and laugh uproariously. Watching people laugh, especially when I didn't know who they were or what they were laughing about.

Suddenly, I felt compelled to do so much and yet nothing at all. Was that the purpose of the exercise? It seemed kind of silly—now that I had discovered some things I loved, I suddenly wanted to do nothing at all.

No sooner did I decide that I wanted to do nothing at all, than I came up with more things I "should" be doing. I should write a note to Janine Giorgenti, thanking her for giving me this opportunity for hope, for showing me a whole different side to life. She had introduced me to alternative medicine. But I ended up not writing the note. I did that a lot. I had all these nice thoughts and things I wanted to do for people, but often never followed through on them. Then I'd beat myself up for not doing it.

So I wondered if I could begin meditating to help calm the persistent thoughts of "things to do." Thinking of it made me want to explore the whole spiritual side of this. I thought I should talk out loud to God and ask for his guidance, help, and strength to stay on the right path and to know which way to go. So, for only the second time in my life, I had a conversation with God. Well, it was really one-sided. He did all the talking.

Just kidding. I asked him to give me the strength to change. To help others, to love more, and to allow love in. To be a better mother and wife and daughter. I asked God to show me the way. To give me a sign and to let this be an opportunity to live a better, happier life, to be a better person. I was learning so much, but would I be able to help others? I'd never asked, "Why me?" or said, "Poor me." Instead, I said, "I know there must be a reason for all this, God. Please guide me to what I'm supposed to be doing."

Even though I hadn't yet left, I was already looking forward to my next trip back to the clinic. I thought it would be best to go for at least a week by myself. It helped me quiet myself. It was a really good feeling to know I didn't have to worry about anything and only had to take care of myself. I was only now beginning to realize just how exhausted I was from my life. Maybe by the time I returned, I would not only have more direction, I would be better able to quiet myself and meditate.

There it was again. I hoped I wasn't being blind and that I really did have that kind of time available—that the cancer wasn't just going to go gangbusters and wipe me out. This was about healing myself, not just medically but mentally and spiritually as well.

One more treatment, a new one: Schwingfeldkabine, also known as SFK. Electromagnetic vibrations were supposed to reestablish order in the diseased parts of the body. I didn't understand it. I actually thought it was a waste of time to sit in a box of metal tubes. But Johan said it was pretty powerful. He told me to imagine light coming in through the base of the skull and traveling throughout the body. I was to put my hands on my legs, palms up. I would imagine taking in all that light. After a while, I was actually in a very peaceful, floating state between waking and sleeping. My hands started to get very hot.

Later that day back in my little apartment, I was thinking about what I had experienced during the SFK. I don't know; there was probably a lot more I could have been doing to help myself spiritually, to be more peaceful and connected to God. I could have found the time to meditate—it was important to be more balanced. I decided that when I returned home, I would cut back on my hours at work. I would try to get closer to a forty- to forty-five-hour work week. I heard the train whistle; my mind had wandered again. The horse-drawn carriage passed by the window again, *clippity clop, clippity clop*. I still hadn't seen it—only heard it. Only in Switzerland.

I did wish the weather were better. It was really cold and raw and had rained every day since we arrived. I had expected a lot more snow—I like snow more than rain—but it was March, so I guess that was to be expected. My headaches started again. It could be the treatments or the fact that I was wearing a turtleneck. It's crazy, but my mother, sister, and I all got headaches from turtlenecks. Kelsey, too. Freaks of nature. So why wear one? Because they looked nice, they were warm, and I always hoped I wouldn't get a headache. The ultimate optimist.

Not all my time was spent at the clinic. Switzerland was in a great geographic location, and there were plenty of places to visit. One day Christian took us to Germany. Imagine that. One minute we were in Switzerland, and an hour later we had our passports checked, took a ferry across Lake Constance, and were in a whole new country, seeing castles. Yes, that's right, really old castles, the kind where knights and kings and queens had lived.

That was all pretty foreign to me (so to speak). In the States, it was a much bigger deal to go to a foreign country. We had Canada and Mexico, but they were still pretty far from New York City. Switzerland, though, was surrounded by interesting countries that were so close by.

While traveling, we stopped at a little café. They had only pastries and cappuccino. (Oh, my God, the pastries looked so good, I was drooling!) So we went to an Italian place. We asked for salads without dressing, and they came covered in oil and vinegar. (Okay, so I have to work on my German a little more.)

Back to work at the clinic again on Monday, I made my second big walk, at Dr. Rau's insistence. He wanted me to walk from the inn to the clinic. It took an hour and a half because I walked at the pace of a turtle and had to stop regularly to rest. I was wiped out, yet it felt so good to have done it. My first big walk had been up the hill near the inn, to see Lake Constance and look over to Austria and Germany. A fifteen-minute walk, and I was looking at two other countries. I think I'm still recovering from that! It was very steep, but every few feet, when I had to stop to catch my breath, there was another spectacular view of mountains or grasslands, all so rich in color. I really thought I could move there.

Biological medicine brought me to a whole new level of learning. It was fascinating to understand just how much of what we do affects our health—most of the time without our knowing it. One area I learned about was dentistry. The clinic had a newly built state-of-the-art building just for dental work. Healthy teeth were important; without them, it was very hard to have a healthy body.

I had never taken very good care of my teeth, as you might have guessed from my fillings on top of fillings. I learned that amalgam fillings, root canals, and infections are extremely detrimental to our health. I learned enough about mercury and root canals to open my eyes. There is a tremendous amount of skepticism around this issue. Hey, I was there, too. Having experienced it myself, though, I became a big believer.

Part of grasping the dentistry required a basic understanding of Chinese acupuncture meridians. The understanding of acupuncture meridians has been around for thousands of years. The treatments can be pretty powerful with the right practitioner. Anyway, the meridians circulate all through the body, including the teeth. Each tooth has meridians that correspond with connected organs or areas in the body.

For example, certain molars rest on the breast meridian. When a root canal, a large amalgam filling, or a crown is placed in or on a tooth, it cuts off or alters the energetic flow. The meridian might correspond to the knees, heart, lungs, or any other area. In fact, in a study of a hundred women with breast cancer, ninety-three of them had undergone root canals on the breast meridian.

Also, root canals continually leak toxins into the body and make people sick. According to some studies, 75 percent of teeth with root canals have residual infections in the dentinal tubules. I'm not a doctor or a scientist, but if I needed a root canal, I'd look into this first. Any type of infection weakens the body and the immune system. There are other options for avoiding root canals. One of the things they do at the clinic is homeopathic injections. Dr. Rau explained that some 75 percent of potential root canals can be avoided with homeopathic injections.

George Meinig's *The Root Canal Cover-up* explains how this is possible. The book details a twenty-five-year study done by Dr. Westin Price and his team of sixty researchers over seventy years ago. He extracted the root canal treated teeth from people with degenerative diseases and placed them under the skin of laboratory animals (usually a rabbit).

In over 5,000 cases, the lab animals developed the same degenerative disease as the patient from whom the tooth was extracted. If the patient had heart disease, the animal developed heart disease. If the patient had kidney disease, the animal developed it, too. If the patient had a problem in the joints, the animal's corresponding joints became involved.

Price explained that some patients would not be affected, because their immune system was strong enough to handle the infection. His statistics showed that about 30 percent of those who had root canals had a strong enough immune system to handle the bacteria and remain in good health. These "healthy" individuals were able to handle it *until* they experienced a severe accident, the flu, a pregnancy, breastfeeding, excessive worry, grief, or some other stress that overwhelmed their immune system, so that they could no longer control the toxins and bacteria coming from the root canal filled tooth. Then they often developed a degenerative disease." This makes sense to me—if we have an ongoing infection anywhere in our body, it is going to challenge our immune system and affect our health.

Sandra, the friend I met from the States, was a striking example of this. She was a young mother who had been experiencing severe pain in her upper jaw. She went to her dentist several times. He kept telling her everything was fine. Any of this sounding familiar? One day, Sandra had trouble breathing and collapsed, unconscious. She was taken to the emergency room, where she was diagnosed with a pleural effusion: fluid in the lung as a result of cancer that had metastasized to the lung. Before that day, she hadn't known she had cancer. The news was grave. She did everything she could in the States, including the raw green diet, and packed her bags for Paracelsus.

On their first or second day, all patients have an appointment with the dentist. In this case, the dentist immediately found a severe infection that had eaten through the bone in Sandra's upper jaw and was approaching her eye socket. The kicker was that it had started in the tooth on the same meridian as the lung. The doctors in the States had been unable to find the primary location of the cancer until she met a doctor who later joined Paracelsus. He had first treated her in the States and identified it as ovarian cancer, which was then confirmed. Unfortunately, this had gone undiagnosed for over a year, even though Sandra had repeatedly told her U.S. doctors that something was wrong in her reproductive area. The infection was removed, and she started to improve.

After root canals comes mercury. Well, I was the poster child for that issue. After I arrived, I had my mercury levels tested—they were literally off the charts. Keep in mind that there are no safe levels of mercury for the human body. It's a deadly toxin, and the Swiss take it very seriously. The people from the company who pick up mercury removed from patients at the clinic wear hazmat suits.

My mercury level was 490. That was after three months of working to detox, so imagine how high it would have been if I had tested before I started to clean myself out. There is no known safe level, but typically it should be below 5. Dr. Rau said the levels were "quite horrible".

I learned that mercury is a neurotoxin that weakens the immune system. It shuts down the white blood cells' ability to process waste. A healthy immune system means a healthy body. When we eat, chew, drink hot liquids, grind our teeth or have mercury fillings put in or drilled out, mercury passes through the soft palate on the roof of the mouth and enters the blood supply. It crosses the blood-brain barrier, affects neurological function, becomes embedded in tissue, and is connected with many diseases.

I had so many of the symptoms, it wasn't funny. Then I heard that mothers pass it on to their children. We had Kelsey tested. Yup, you guessed it: her levels were also very high. I had passed it to her transplacentally, and it passes to the fetus at an accelerated rate. How else could a three-year-old have such high levels? Talk about guilt. Two parents with cancer, a congenital brain hemorrhage, and now mercury poisoning. That sucked! Poor kid.

I hadn't had any root canals, but I did have an infection on the tooth corresponding to the breast meridian. There were also amalgams that took up pretty much the whole tooth. So I figured I would go one step further. When mom came over, I took her straight to the dentist. She had spinal stenosis, severe arthritis in her hip and knee, and a problem with a drop foot. You guessed it: she'd had root canals on those meridians.

I heard it again and again from patient after patient. Many of them experienced problems on the meridians where they'd had root canals and amalgams. I received lots of confirmation that this was for real. It went back to biological medicine: get to the root cause of why illness happened, get rid of the cause, and give the body a chance to build itself back up again.

The impact of mercury and root canals wasn't always accurate, because some patients had stronger immune systems. But if something is accurate most of the time, it's worth looking into. Why take the chance of hurting ourselves unnecessarily? Why not do *everything we can* to ensure our good health?

After all the fascinating knowledge I gained, and the extensive treatments, it was time to head back to reality. I loaded up with supplements and instructions for what to do until my next trip to the clinic, four months away. Once home, I went back to work and put my new program into action. It combined what I had done and learned at the clinic with what I had gotten from Richard and Mary. I continued diligently on the path. There was hope!

Chapter Sixteen

A Ray of Sunshine Peeks through the Clouds: My Second Trip to Switzerland

I returned to the clinic in July, a beautiful time in Switzerland. The schedule was very full because this visit was shorter. At my first hyperthermia, I reached 103.8, which was great. I wanted to go higher, but the infusion needle was difficult to bear. They also gave me glutathione, powerful stuff against cancer. Still no emotional experiences, though. Was I pathetic, or what?

I had the opportunity to work with a new doctor. He covered a lot of areas and was very knowledgeable and insightful, especially on emotional issues. One of the things he did was neural therapy, which could be painful but was very effective. It was done to my lungs and throat.

I didn't like that very much. Between the trouble with swallowing after neural therapy, a bad cold, hyperthermia, and a lack of sleep from coughing, I felt the worst I had ever felt at Paracelsus. Although in some ways it was a vacation from life, it wasn't really a vacation. At times, it was really hard work—the work of regaining my health—but still a job I gladly took on.

* * *

On a happier note, I had one of my most memorable experiences that trip. The day was sunny and the sky a gorgeous blue. I went up past Appenzell and did a hike with Tina, another American friend. Okay, so it took almost the whole day to do what someone else could have done in an hour or two, but I did it!

It was extremely difficult to walk and hike. The mountains were steep and rocky, even though we were on a path. I honestly didn't think I would make it. My legs were shaking so much, I was afraid to take the next step. I had to keep stopping to catch my breath. I actually saw a helicopter medevac a cow off the mountain, and secretly wished I could get a lift back down, too!

I honestly don't think I've ever seen anything so beautiful. It was like being in a dream. Sometimes I asked myself if I really was aware of how spectacular it all was. Once we made it to the top, we stopped and ate lunch overlooking a breathtaking turquoise lake. We got some fresh goat's milk from a farmer who stopped us during the hike. He was thrilled. I'm not big on goat's milk. That may be because I was allergic to so many things as a child, and so sick all the time, that the only thing I could keep down was goat's milk. I had overdosed on it early.

This kind man also showed us how he milked the cows—all without our speaking a word of German, or his speaking a word of English. He chattered on as he worked, though, having the time of his life. He squirted milk all over the place and at us just for kicks. We laughed so hard, I had to sit down.

Ah, the simple life. I felt a huge sense of accomplishment at making it up there. It's one of the most memorable places I have ever been, and all the more so for my having made it up there. It made me miss Kelsey and Kevin, though, and I couldn't wait to take them up when they came. Next time, I would go up by cable car!

The next day was another happy day. I was sitting—lounging, actually—on the side of a hill on the Wanderweg, just beside the Schützengarten, listening to dogs bark; cows moo; church bells, cow bells, and goat bells ring; children play; and trains whistle. There went that horse-drawn carriage! I did all this under the most glorious blue sky. What could have been better?

Unfortunately, this luxury had to end. I had chores and work to do, which I dreaded. I couldn't help but ask, "Why am I doing this? Why not just lie here and screw the rest?" Nope, gotta work, work, work. I had to clean vegetables, make juice and soup, clean the apartment, do some wash, write e-mails, and do some work from the office. All I really wanted to do was lie there for the rest of the afternoon and read my mindless novel on this spectacular mountainside, basking in the sun. Wow! I could add that to the list of things I loved to do!

I made another friend, named Kathleen Muto. She was from the States and had moved to work in the Paracelsus Clinic as a dental hygienist. Imagine the guts that took. She created this awesome opportunity for herself. She worked four days and took off the other three to visit other countries on the weekends. It wasn't any big deal for her to hop on the train with her bicycle or take a plane to another country.

I would have loved to do that. I thought maybe we could home-school Kelsey for a year and do it. Kevin just rolled his eyes.

Kathleen was a sweetheart, the kind of person you love right off the bat. We shopped for some things for her new apartment. Then she invited me over for an awesome dinner. It sure was nice to have a friend there. It turned out that Kathleen was not only a good friend but the best dental hygienist I've ever come across. She was incredibly thorough and knowledgeable and had some cleaning techniques I've never experienced in the States.

By the third trip, with me relentlessly torturing Dr. Rau about the benefits of the raw green diet, he saw how well I was doing, and was beginning to believe that raw foods really do work. He admitted that if he were ever diagnosed with cancer, he would eat raw for the first few months and then go strictly alkaline—along with all the other treatments, of course. This was a huge breakthrough, to have him agree with the effectiveness of a mainly vegetable-based diet and they have since adopted it at the clinic.

Mom joined me for this trip. We stayed at the clinic for one week. The second week, we went with Dr. Rau to a retreat at Paracelsus's sister clinic in Al Ronc. It was in the southern part of Switzerland, the Italian-speaking part—yeah, now we're talkin', baby! I got to use some of those "*ciao bella's*" and "*bellisima's*" and "*andiamo's*" (which means "let's go"—one of my favorite words).

Unfortunately, every time I tried to speak Italian, some German, Spanish, French, or a combination of the four came out instead. I couldn't help but think, *I'm in Italy.* That's the one crazy part of being in Switzerland: you really think you're in a country other than Switzerland. In the German-speaking part, I thought I was in Germany. In the Italian-speaking part, I thought I was in Italy. I couldn't wait to visit the French-speaking part.

Kevin called to tell me what Kelsey had said on the way home from the airport: "Poor Mommy has to go all the way to Switzerland by herself with no husband and little girl. Poor, poor Mommy."

Kevin had said, "Well, Granny is with her."

"Poor, poor Mommy and Granny have to go all the way to Switzerland by themselves with no husband and little girl. Poor, poor Mommy and Granny."

She was so cute! I missed her so much. That was one of the toughest parts about being there.

Now, I know I told you the Swiss-German part was magnificent. But the southern section was breathtaking! The clinic was more like a self-contained spa overlooking spectacular snow-covered mountains and a valley. That, and they spoke Italian. Better yet, we could juice blood oranges! Ever juiced blood oranges? Oh, my God!

Much of the treatments in Al Ronc were the same as in the main clinic. The difference was that here you stayed on site, which made life easier. The other difference was that Dr. Rau wasn't at this clinic all the time—he would mainly come down for the intensive weeks, such as this one. I had one of my most memorable moments in Al Ronc when I met Leena Nicolaou. Leena taught about colonics and colon health. That's right: "How well do you poop?"

One day she worked with me on a coffee enema. I climbed onto a table on my hands and knees. My arse (as we of Irish heritage may politely call it) in the air, exposed to the open door and hung out for the world to see.

Rather shyly, I said, "Uh, Leena?"

"Yes?"

"Uh, the door is open."

"Yes?" As though it was the most logical thing for the door to be doing at that moment and as if I had been very silly to mention it.

"Well, maybe we should close it."

She waved her arm and said, "Oh, if someone comes by, tell them to go away, that you are enjoying your coffee."

She swept out of the room as I burst out laughing—not the best thing to do in the middle of an enema. That was just about one of the best laughs I have ever had. She was so awesome. I just loved her. I guess we Americans really were too modest.

While in Al Ronc, I started to cough. Now, this wasn't any old cough that could be treated with over-the-counter syrup in a week. This was a cough from having radiation to my lungs. Real nasty. The kind that never let up. It was unproductive and exhausting. Many times, I coughed so hard and for so long, I threw up.

No one could have prepared me for the real impact. They might have said, "You may develop a cough." Okay, but they hadn't said it was the kind you couldn't catch your breath from, that wouldn't let you sleep, and that you couldn't soothe no matter what—or that it is much worse in the cold air. *Oh, and by the way, it might last a year or, come to think of it, your lifetime.* They didn't mention any of those things.

Oh, yeah, and did I mention the pain that started in the whole upper left side of my body while I was walking in the mountains? It was an albatross from then on. And did I mention that my ribs popped out of place, too? Yup, that was also from the radiation. I turned my head, and two of my ribs popped right out from my spine. Talk about excruciating.

It was like having broken ribs. It was unbearably painful to breathe or move. And if that weren't bad enough, there was the sickening pain when I laughed or coughed. And what was I experiencing? A chronic cough. Not a good combo. My ribs popped out three times.

It seemed that just after it would get somewhat better, I would move the wrong way and it happened again. Each time, the severe pain lasted several months. The extensive radiation had burned the nerves, muscles, and tissue so severely they had adhered to my bones, so whenever one part of me moved, the whole kit and caboodle moved.

If I lay on my left side, I wheezed. I had numbness and tingling in my arm and hand, and I lost much of the movement in my left arm. I couldn't lift it or use it for most normal functions. And the pain when I did move it was often not worth it. Any type of exercise caused the most excruciating pain.

When they performed the second round of surgeries and radiation, it burned the nerve endings and made them even more hyperstimulated. To this day, I have constant pain. I can't bear to have anyone touch my arm, side, chest, or stomach. You'd think damaged nerves would be numb, but for some reason, just the opposite happens. Like phantom pain in a limb that has been amputated.

Ever tried to scratch an itch after getting Novocain at the dentist? That's what it's like for me all the time. I have itches under the skin that I can't scratch. Did I mention these were all side effects from chemo and radiation? Thank you, radiation! Thank you, chemo! That and my heart. Yes, my heart was within range of the radiation. I try not to think about the damage done to it—I don't want it to break.

It didn't matter how bad things seemed. The bottom line was that I was alive, and I believed that one day I would find a way to heal all those issues. The key was that I hadn't let anything stop me. Other things about me were good and were working just fine. Even if it was only my mind or my breath or my smile or my eyes, or moving my big toe, or that I had the ability to pee—now, that's a good one. It would really have sucked not to be able to pee.

I loved Switzerland and Paracelsus. The clinic was awesome, an amazing experience, and very effective. Everything is what you make of it. What you put out, you get back. If you put out anger, you get back anger. If you put out resentment and fear, you get back resentment and fear. If you put out distrust, you get back distrust from others and more reasons not to trust. If you look for things to go wrong, you will find more than enough things going wrong.

Much more importantly, though, if you put out good things, you get back good things. If you look for good things, you will find more than enough good things. If you look for things that make you happy, you will find more than enough things to make you happy. If you look for the good in people, you will find more than enough good people.

Your experiences will be determined by how you look at them. I chose to look at all that happened to us as a blessing. I look forward to going back to Paracelsus again one day. The only thing I would do differently is to make sure I stay with the green diet. That's when I've had the best results.

Chapter Seventeen

WHERE THE FUN PICKS UP:
THE AMAZING VOYAGE
OUT OF CANCER

I can't point to a specific moment when I made the decision that made my being alive possible. I do know what the decision was, though. The most important decision I have made in my life was to say, *No, I don't accept your diagnosis. I'll do whatever it takes. I'll do it all.* And the first thing I did was to *choose to live!*

Since the change in diet, the supplements, the alternative treatments, and my choice to live, nine years have gone by, and Kevin and I are cancer free. Now, tell me that's not freakin' *awesome!*

One of my happiest days was when Dr. Rau was looking at my blood in a training seminar when I began studying biological medicine. I just had to learn more about it. I know, I know: from Wall Street to biological medicine? What crazy thing was she up to now? I just couldn't help myself. I was giddy with excitement, bursting to share with others just how powerful biological medicine, raw foods, an "alkaline" lifestyle, and microscopy were—and not just for cancer but for all sorts of illnesses and ailments. I thought of all the people all over the world who were just accepting everyday ailments *and* debilitating life-threatening disease as their fate, as if there were nothing they could do to heal themselves. And I knew, in my heart and in my gut—and now also in my head—that there were more options open to them, *to us all.* I had to learn more about it. I realized how many people were living as I had been. Daily they endured aches and pains, depression, anxiety, brain fog, digestive problems, headaches, allergies, blemishes, extra pounds, and just plain old *exhaustion,* all the while taking all kinds of over-the-counter and prescription medicines to keep the symptoms at bay—but *never getting rid of the cause*! Once I knew what it was like to feel great in just thirty days after living my whole life feeling lousy, I couldn't imagine going back to the way I had felt before. I couldn't imagine not sharing what I had discovered with others so that they, too, could go from feeling "just okay," mediocre, or lousy to feeling great, too.

Anyway, back to Dr. Rau. I had volunteered to be the cancer example for him and have my blood shown on the big screen to teach the other students. He was going to show them the signs of degeneration to look for when a patient had cancer. You can't actually *see* the cancer cells, but you can see the environment that the cancer thrives in. I had just finished back-to-back trips to Paracelsus and Hippocrates Health Institute, a raw-food holistic health center in West Palm Beach, Florida.

He looked at the blood, then to me, then back to the blood, then back to me with this incredulous look on his face. He was astonished. The blood looked *too good*. I was supposed to be the cancer example, but he couldn't find any of the degenerative signs. So I became something much better. In his heavy German accent, Dr. Rau said, "Well, ladies and gentlemen, Mrs. O'Brien's blood is an example of how *healthy* blood looks and why biological medicine works." (Yes, he still called me "Mrs. O'Brien.") At first, I was just as astonished as he, and then I was beaming! *Woo-hoo!*

I loved going back to my oncologist after that, because she was so encouraging. She would look at me and say, "Just keep doing whatever you're doing. I don't want to know what it is, but you're a miracle. You're doing something right. Don't screw it up."

When she stopped practicing, a few years after my initial stage 4 diagnosis, I switched to a third oncologist. I really liked her, too. Our first meeting was really funny. Mom was by my side, as usual. The doctor looked down at the records, then at me. She was perplexed as she flipped through my records again very thoroughly several times. She looked up at me with concern and asked very seriously, "Is there some kind of mistake in the records? The reports all show that you were diagnosed with stage 4 cancer five years ago, but there's no indication of it anywhere."

I said, "No, there is no mistake. I *had* stage four cancer."

She was visibly taken aback. "Are you sure?"

"Yes," I chuckled, "I'm sure"

"Do you have any idea how lucky you are?" she asked. "You're a miracle."

"Thank you."

"But … do you *really* know how lucky you are?"

"Yes, I know. I am very blessed." I smiled as gratitude washed over me.

She turned to my mother. "Do *you* have any idea how lucky she is?"

"Yes!" Mom said, grinning from ear to ear.

"Just keep doing whatever you're doing," the oncologist said. She kept repeating herself, saying, "This is miraculous. Do you know how lucky you are?"

"Yes, I do! Thank you!"

I did a little happy dance in my mind, said, *Thank you, God!* and gave God a high five.

The oncologist I chose to work with after I was diagnosed with stage 4 never would give me a prognosis. She didn't believe in them, and I think she's right. If your doctor pronounces a death sentence, how else can you have hope? If I had been told I had six to twelve months to live, that sounds pretty final to me. It would have put more fear in me. It's all I would have thought about.

Being told there was nothing they could do to save me had been bad enough. But if they had told me I had only six months, based on what I now know about thoughts and feelings creating reality, I would have reacted very differently. I probably would have said, "Okay, I have six months, so why eat vegetables? I'm having filet mignon covered in merlot sauce, and greasy burgers and triple fudge cake." Or, worse, I would have set that date and then spiraled into a deep depression, feeding the cancer all it wanted. Or, knowing me, I would have 'worked' to tie up all the loose ends, especially for my daughter.

And if I had gotten the prognosis and done those things, you wouldn't be reading this, and I wouldn't be here.

You see, I would have been in a *dying* frame of mind instead of a *living* frame of mind. In healing myself, I realized just how important it was to stay in this living frame of mind. It moved me forward, kept me searching, kept me strong, and kept me believing that it was possible to live!

If I had stayed in the dying frame of mind, I wouldn't have thought I had enough time for anything else to work, and I would have stuck with the chemo to prolong my life a little, regardless of the *quality* of that life. Had I made those choices, I am 100 percent certain I would not be here now.

Instead, I have years and years to *live*, free of cancer and free of fear— although the fear, in some ways, was beneficial. The fear of stage 4 cancer drove me to action, but I had the benefit of not having a deadline on my life. No one should ever put a stopwatch on anyone's life—it only tricks us into counting down instead of using each day proactively.

Not being given a prognosis was essential, but family support really carried us through. My family and friends were amazing. They were terrified at times, and God knows they didn't always agree with my decisions, but they stuck by me and did all they could to help.

My sister Kathy and my sister-in-law Barbara spent untold hours learning how to make the food on our approved "yes" list, and there hasn't been a holiday or family event yet in which they haven't had something for me to eat. And no loved one has ever tried to get me to eat something that wasn't healthy just because I was losing too much weight.

Kathy came over at the drop of a hat, even though she lived forty-five minutes away. She and our friend Jackie decorated the house inside and out for Christmas and, with my friend Jen, helped me get rid of a small mountain of clutter. My mom, my brother Rob and sister-in-law Naomi, my friend Diane, and my brother Rich and sister-in-law Barbara watched Kelsey whenever needed. They made sure I could travel worry free to Switzerland and Hippocrates Health Institute. My sister-in-law Patty flew in from Michigan anytime we needed anything, and even when we didn't she would ask when she could come and help out.

Kevin's mom, Kathleen, who has always been a ray of sunshine, would come out for days at a time to help us, full of enthusiasm, with a joke, tickles for Kelsey, and prayer chains from the ladies at church. Always upbeat and encouraging, she would tell me how terrific I was for the way I just took this challenge on—encouragement that I really needed to hear during the toughest days, when I wasn't feeling all that terrific. Rich, my ever-generous brother, always made sure we were okay financially, my dad and my brother Rob fixed whatever needed fixing around the house, and my friend Pam dropped off bags of washed vegetables for us to juice. My cousin Linda sent me a piece of Padre Pio's robe and a very special statue of him, and another friend, Mary, sent us Swiss francs and a rosary ring. Friends and family would slip quietly in and out as I slept for hours at a time on the chaise, unaware that they had even been there. My friends Trish and Jen joined me on the journey, matching my excitement for each new thing I learned, so that I never felt alone—which can easily happen when you're sailing on uncharted waters.

Instead of asking, "What can I do?" people just looked around, saw what needed doing, and did it. When someone asks, "What can I do?" the natural reply is, "Nothing, that's okay." It's harder to ask for help than to say thanks for an unasked favor. One of the most humbling things I have had to learn is to receive and to allow others to give. I learned that many people want to help and that saying no can be hurtful. I had never looked at it that way, but in the same way that I had always wanted to give, others did, too. But I must tell you, accepting help was a tough one for me at first. Then I realized that my survival depended on it.

And there were all the prayers, cards, and calls. There is power in prayer, and it sure felt good to know we had prayer groups cheering for us. We were on my mother-in-law, Kathleen's, church prayer group for so long, they must finally have said, "Jeez, Louise! Aren't these two either dead or alive and kickin' by now?" The cards and calls helped us know that people cared. They were sending good intentions, even from people we didn't know, and there is powerful energy in that. I am all the more grateful when I think that there are people who don't have anyone. I can't imagine what it would be like to have gone through this without any support.

For me, getting well was really a series of decisions and listening to guidance—punctuated by miracles, to be sure, but it was the decisions and actions that made those miracles possible.

Let's face it: if you start cleaning yourself out and building your immune system, the very first thing you do might add one minute to your life. The second thing you do might add five minutes. Add a different way of helping yourself, and you might add an hour. Be consistent, and before you know it, you've added a day, a week, and then a year. Keep going, and you have five years. Next thing you know, you could have a complete *shift* in your entire biological structure. Then guess what? The cancer is gone and you feel great! It could happen on the first day or the thousandth day. No one knows. But Kevin and I are proof that it can happen.

Miracles happen every day. I can trace my miracles back to a three-step process, which may work for you or someone you know. It's simple. (But note that "simple" doesn't mean "easy."). So … ready? Here it is:

1. Think about what it is you *really* want. Spend some time on this so you're satisfied that this is it, without a doubt.

2. Now, ASK FOR IT!

3. Okay, now you've done it—you've just opened the "miracles" door. Now be open to receive answers and guidance on your next steps. Once you do open up to it, I truly believe you will be given that guidance.

There are some other things I learned that can make healing easier. For one, it helps to look at healing as a process, not a magic bullet. And it's crucially important that we look at it from the perspective of healing our whole being: body, mind *and* spirit. It's like a three-legged stool—leave any one of the legs off, and it's not going to stand. I truly, deeply believe that the importance of healing at an emotional and spiritual level is seriously overlooked and has a dramatic impact on our success.

A support system is another one of the keys to success. Anything family and friends can do in a positive way is *awesome*. And one of the most important things they can do is to be supportive. If you have someone close to you who is ill, make sure that you are coming from a loving, caring place with the best of intentions. No matter how painful it is for you and how hard it might be, you can be of tremendous help just by supporting their choices—even if you don't agree with them.

Another thing Kevin and I know from personal experience is that we aren't helping the person who is ill by letting them feel sorry for themselves. For a short while, okay, fine—releasing emotions is important—but if it's prolonged, it won't help. Healing those emotions is essential, though. You might need to gently encourage action. After all, no one wants to be told what to do, especially when they are terrified or feel lousy. You have the ability to carry them, walk by their side, or let them fall.

It's not helpful to say, "Oh, it's so hard to eat that way—all those vegetables. Yuck, you're going to turn green! Can't you eat some pasta or a cheeseburger or some regular food? It'll make you feel better." That kind of "support" doesn't really help. In fact, you could actually be *hurting* them. Feeding them ice cream, weight-gain drinks, or other unhealthy things just to keep weight on also feeds the cancer.

Give them all the support they need so they can feed their body with positive thoughts and foods that will heal instead of hurt. Take really good care of them and love them with all that you have, but don't treat them as if they were dying. It's not going to help them if everyone around them is coming from a place of fear and condolence.

If the doctors say something negative that is not going to put them in a *living* frame of mind, you can make a choice to ignore it. Emotions, especially negative ones, have a powerful energetic force. Now I'm really going to go out on a limb. You may think I'm nuts (okay, so maybe the thought has already occurred to you), but give it a try anyway. Send them healing energy; don't send them dying energy. Treat them as if they are not just living but healing and growing more vibrant.

Do a meditation or visualization for them. Imagine them being healed by a vacuum suctioning out all the harmful things through the top of their head. Then fill them with a green healing light that makes them stronger. Ask whatever higher power you believe in to surround them and fill them with beautiful, healing white light.

We all need to be surrounded by positive energy. Don't you feel better around uplifting people? I do. I call them "the *swirl*." The people you love to be with, who inspire you and make you want to swirl around and dance inside and out. They surround you and engulf you with their swirl of good energy and feelings. We all need to be surrounded by that positive energy.

We do need that time of mourning, though. Mourning for things lost. Then know when it's time to pick yourself up and take control. Know when it's time to say, "I don't care what the doctors say. *I'm* in control of my destiny, not the doctors." Say, "I am healthy!"

It isn't easy. Maybe it's really hard, but isn't it worth it? Whatever the outcome, isn't it better to spend every possible minute of whatever time we have on this planet in a state of mind working toward positive things than to live in negativity? That's a whole lot better than feeling miserable. What benefit is there to feeling negative?

We hear all the time that everything is energy and, moreover, that like attracts like. This is really cool because it means that if our thoughts are energy, then good thoughts attract good things. It's not really a great big *secret* anymore, right? So if you can have a positive thought that serves you and will help attract what you want, why bother hanging out in negative thoughts that have harmful effects? Why would anyone consciously attract negative things into their life?

Can you imagine a newborn baby feeling depressed or "not good enough"? No way! They are on the top of the world. Just look at how happy they are! Why is everyone so magnetically attracted to babies? It's because they feel so good, their happiness is contagious. What's the first thing you do when you see a baby? You try to make them smile. We act like ding-a-lings, making all those funny faces to get that smile.

Another great way to keep those cancer-free juices going and feel great is to *dance.* I'm not kidding—shake those hips! It sounds ridiculously simple, but when you put on a song that really makes you want to shake that booty (and, by the way, the crazier the better), a little silliness comes out and raises all those great brain chemicals that make you feel good!

In our family, we do it all the time! Kevin got a little bummed one day with a project that wasn't panning out. He sat down on the couch and was just kind of staring off into space, but clearly not in a happy place. The stereo was on, and I pulled him up by his hands and started to dance with him. He was like a sack of potatoes at first, shoulders slumped and with a little pouty face on, but the longer I danced with him (probably a minute) and the more I made him shake his hips, the more he relaxed and had to fight not to smile. And when Kelsey came over and squeezed in between us like the filling in a sandwich (just as she has done ever since she was a toddler whenever she sees us hugging or dancing), then he couldn't help but smile.

Next thing we knew, we all were dancing and laughing—Kelsey and I, Kelsey and Kevin, Kevin and I. Kevin said, "I'm better now." The whole thing took less than two minutes, and the whole house was happy again.

That's how easy it can be! Happy thoughts are inextricably connected to happy movement—give it a try!

Understandably, it stinks to have your whole life changed in an instant. But what if that change turns out to the best thing that ever happened, as it did for Kevin and me? What would stink far more would be to look back and say, "I wish I had done something different."

If we feel sorry for ourselves and stay in a negative place, how can we let in all the good things that are meant to come our way? And I'm not talking just about feeling sorry for ourselves if we have cancer here. This applies to the rest of our lives, too. We seem to be wired to look for what's going wrong and how to "fix" it, instead of looking for what's going *right*. When we focus on things going right, the universe tends to accommodate us and send us more things to go right, plain and simple!

And if we also say, *I'll do whatever it takes,* the universe will often send what we need. I really believe that. The key is to be open to it and then take action. *Hope with action.*

Sure, I live with limitations. But I counter them by thinking of the greatest gift I've ever received: my life! A gift beyond measure. I say, "One day I will move my arm again! One day I will do a cartwheel. One day I will live without physical pain and limitation." I really believe I will find a way to recover from those things, just as I have done with everything else. I will swim again! Ski again! Golf again! I will run and jump and play again!

Why do I think I can? Because I tell myself I can. It's just a matter of focusing and being open. I believe that this can happen. And if not, what have I lost? Wasted a few good vibes and positive thoughts? I can live with that. At least I tried and felt good about it instead of feeling down. There's certainly something good about that.

And the same is possible for all of us. If I could make these lifestyle changes, especially given my horrific diet history and challenges, anyone with the right resources can make them, too. Even if changing your life doesn't do everything you want it to do, could taking on the challenge be worse than giving up and succumbing to despair? This is what we really want: to live a healthy life while feeling great—isn't it?

Chapter Eighteen

THE SUN IS SHINING:
MIRACLES BIG AND SMALL

O kay, you've probably been wondering when I would finally get to this part, the next fascinating step of our journey. I can't pinpoint the moment it began, the moment when a whole new world began to open up for me—a world that I was aware of but hadn't begun to fathom. I know. Here she goes again. No, don't say it. No, not that! Not … *spiritual*." Yes, spiritual! There! It's all out on the table now.

So I can't pinpoint the exact moment I began the spiritual part of my journey, but, wow, has it been powerful! I mean, obviously, you have to believe that we were being guided and that there was a bigger plan, a "big picture." You really can't just make this stuff up. The more and more I am aware of it, the more I glimpse the power behind so much of what has happened. Somewhere along our physical and emotional roads, I began to question the spiritual power. I'm not sure if it was the day Kevin had his brain hemorrhage and I felt his deceased dad sit down next to me on the bed, or the day I had my powerful experience with Padre Pio. Maybe it was the day *The Celestine Prophecy* jumped out at me from among the hundreds of other books on my friend's bookshelf and opened me up to a whole new world. It might even have happened the day I learned I was "going to die."

I began to question my purpose on this earth and asked myself what I had really accomplished. Things happened—undeniable things that made me crave more experiences like the one at San Giovanni Rotondo and finding

Janine Giorgenti, the talented suit designer who introduced me to alternative medicine. Coincidences? I don't think so.

Some of the spiritual journey progressed without my even being aware of it, and I can see it only now, in hindsight. But I know this: there is a much higher power out there, and I have a strong desire to be connected with it. I always felt a strong relationship and connection to God, but this was different. I may not have been terribly in tune with it, but I knew there was something more out there, and it fascinated me. And I grew daily more and more aware of things that were beyond me.

I wanted to get closer to God. I wanted the serenity of the Buddhist monks. I wanted to stop guessing about things and just *know.* I wanted to be more in tune with the guidance I was so obviously getting. I wanted to quiet my mind, raise my consciousness. I wanted a direct connection to the divine. A way to believe in myself, love myself, and stop beating myself up over anything and everything. I wanted to realize that I did, in fact, have value.

When I started to look for those things, the next turning point appeared. I was lying in bed, in despair. Sometimes I didn't stop to *feel* anymore. I was in a "doing" mode, on autopilot. I had made it through what many people couldn't. I had survived. Other people might have given up, but I hadn't. I had accomplished something tremendous just by living.

So what was I still missing? I knew there must be more to life than what I had. I kept telling myself, *I should be elated. I was supposed to be dead, but I'm alive!* Right? So why did I still feel that nagging, that sadness, that empty feeling of something missing, that feeling of being lost? There had to be something more. I got down on my knees to pray. (Remember what happened the last time I did that? It put me on this course that, undeniably, saved my life, so you have to figure something good might come of it again, right?)

Okay, God, I said, *I know there's more to life than this. I know that if it's out there, you will show me the way. So please, God, help me. Show me the way.*

Now, I wasn't expecting an angel to jump into the water, as Clarence did in *It's a Wonderful Life,* but two days later I got *the* phone call from Richard.

"Joyce, there's something I want to share with you and Kevin."

I was skeptical, but it was Richard. He had put me on the path that saved my life, and as a scientist, he had never recommended something unless it was tried and true and proven. Much as the first time I had spoken to him, I didn't understand a word he was saying. I didn't *hear* the message the first time. God was giving me the answer to my prayer the same way he had the first time I spoke to Richard—only this time, I was listening.

He told Kevin and me about a weekend training that he and Mary had just finished, called Personal Dynamics. They felt that it had opened up a whole new world for them. More than anything, it cleared away much of the emotional baggage that had been holding them back. It had also given them more peace and clarity.

I was skeptical, but I knew I needed some of that, and I knew enough to trust Richard. Kevin was adamantly opposed. If it smacked of self-improvement, he wanted no part of it. He feared change, feared seeing his own limitations, and, even more than that, feared his own potential. As he put it, he wanted to stay in his own "safe little box." He liked that box. It was comfortable, and he knew it well. He didn't care if something better waited just outside.

Poor guy never stood a chance. Silly him, he married me, and I *love* change!

Kevin wanted no part of it, but he finally agreed that our lives could be better, less cluttered, and less stressful.

The training was a combination of lecture and experiential activities in which the participants (that's us) are actively engaged. Kevin was so resistant, he wanted to leave after the first day, and again after the second. Seriously, he sat there with his arms crossed, clearly agitated. I thought he might bolt any second. But by the end of the third day, a major shift had happened for him, and he couldn't wait to go back the next morning. All I wanted was sleep, and he wanted to show up early. Ugh! "Go away," I groaned from under the pillow. Just as with the diet and blood work during our second visit with Richard and Mary, he was getting more out of this than I was, and with less effort.

Much of the training was based on getting rid of the blockages that stop us from having whatever we want in our lives. Blockages come from belief systems that we picked up, whether from parents, teachers, or life, that cause us to think in a particular way. The training was geared toward releasing blockages from emotional traumas and healing painful memories, from childhood all the way up to present. It's sobering how childhood memories that seem as if they couldn't possibly still affect us can embed painful traumas so deeply that they form a part of our belief system and affect us as adults. The training taught us how to see these disempowering belief systems for what they are, and then to look at ourselves and life in a way that empowered us.

For example, the thought that *I'm not good enough* might come from a parent, teacher, older sibling, other kids, or grandparents—perhaps with the best of intentions—telling you that you weren't good at something. It could be the pain of a bad experience. Childhood abuse in any form, for example, can cause you to put up walls against intimate relationships. Trust issues could result from a hurt received from someone you loved or trusted, including friends and siblings. Our need to control might come from things being out of control when we were kids. A fear holding us back from accomplishing what we really want to do or have might come from a trauma as a child.

The exercises started us on a whole new path of clearing the emotional experiences that made us feel bad inside—the ones that create that inner chatter that makes us feel inadequate. It was about taking responsibility, forgiving, letting go, and taking action.

Kevin and I are so much more in tune with each other that we really never disagree strongly anymore. If we do have a disagreement now, it lasts no more than five minutes, because we each recognize where the other is coming from, take responsibility quickly, and move past it.

The training wasn't the solution to every problem, but it was really powerful and did provide us with an awareness, a way to look at things differently. It catapulted us into a whole new world. It made us much more aware of our thoughts and feelings, the words that create our reality, and how those words affect others. It helped jump-start our realization that we were limiting ourselves by allowing these beliefs to exist. Yes, sometimes it can be that simple. Sometimes just recognizing and then changing the way we think can improve our lives dramatically.

The training showed me how to forgive others easily but, more importantly, to forgive myself.

Negative self-talk hurts us deeply, and yet, we don't realize how much it affects our lives and those around us. If each of us worked on our pain and our limiting beliefs and took responsibility for what we are creating, this world would be a much better place. There would be a huge reduction in crime, war, divorce, disease, child abuse, drug and alcohol abuse—all the things that happen when we hold on to the mistaken beliefs we have held since childhood.

I just can't help but tell people about the training. Several of my friends have said it allowed them to repair relationships and save marriages. One friend even met her future husband there.

I let go of a huge burden of clutter in my head and my house. I cleaned out half the stuff in our house, accomplishing in a short time what would have taken me months to do in the past.

We went to Disney World right afterward, and I had more fun than when I went as a kid. In fact, I was elated. The three of us raced each other to the rides and had a blast. (Well, okay, Kevin and Kelsey raced and then ran around chasing each other until I caught up).

It was truly awesome to see Kevin's tremendous growth as a person. Not that he was half bad before, mind you, but he became much happier and more balanced, more open, more spiritual, and more outwardly focused. He says he is thrilled that he stepped outside his comfy little box into a whole new and exciting world, to a path that we could now travel together. So a life-changing experience is possible for anyone.

This was the best part: I no longer felt that despair, that emptiness. I knew I was on the right path. It was as if someone had taken an eraser and wiped my internal slate clean of things that were harmful to me emotionally. The cancerous thoughts and feelings had been removed, and I felt fifty pounds lighter. A light was turned on inside me, allowing me to feel good about myself in a way I never had before. I felt like a kid again. It was the happiest I had ever been in my entire life. *Phew!* Glad to be rid of all that junk that could have overflowed a landfill!

Personal Dynamics was just the first step on a path of personal growth that continues to transform our lives and our health to higher and higher levels. We have since attended other trainings (as opposed to seminars, where you just sit and listen). Trainings are more effective because they are experiential, life-changing, and because you are involved as an active participant. For me, that's the best way to learn. When I live it, I really get it.

Once again, I just needed to ask and I was guided. That was really the starting point of our emotional and spiritual healing. From there, many other things opened up for us because *we* opened up.

So I continued on my path to find my life's purpose. I opened myself to yoga and meditation and many other things the universe offered. My desire to reach a higher spiritual level burned stronger and stronger. I became so much more aware that the energy I put out came back to me.

Without even knowing about it, much of what I had been doing throughout my journey was based on the principles of *The Secret* and Abraham Hicks. Essentially, it's the law of attraction: our thoughts and feelings create our reality. It goes way beyond the power of positive thinking and opens up a whole new world.

When I saw *The Secret* for the first time, I sat on the edge of my seat, quite literally. I was so excited, I could barely sit still to watch the ending. I ran to the phone to call my friend Tricia, who had told me I *had* to watch the movie, which was released only the week before. "This is unbelievable!" I told her. "It's freakin' awesome. It makes perfect sense. This is insane that it's what I've been doing all along without knowing it, good *and* bad." I mean, really, who the heck wants to attract a few rounds of cancer and a brain hemorrhage? But then again, it was the same natural law in action when I attracted the amazing, lifesaving, and life-altering things that have completely transformed my health, my career, my path, my relationships, my future—my whole life!—and opened me up to all this rockin' spiritual stuff. These principles had been instrumental in attracting the things I needed to survive. I had always believed I would live—I just needed guidance on how to do it. The only thing still holding me back was my negative self-talk, and even that was something I was so aware of after the trainings that I often caught myself and shifted.

Something powerful continued to nag at me, though. I still wasn't clear about my reason for being on this planet—my life purpose. I needed to know I wasn't wasting my time, to know that I would never look back at my life with regret over not accomplishing the things I was meant to accomplish. I knew I wanted to help others so they wouldn't have to go through what Kevin and I had gone through. But it was so much more than that—I wanted to make a difference; I just didn't know what that looked like.

So again I prayed for a few days and asked God to help me. A couple of days later, the message arrived loud and clear. It started as a whisper and got louder and louder until it was booming too loud to ignore. I kept hearing it day after day. Was it God? I think so. I do know that it was coming from a much higher source than my own little mind and ego. It was unmistakable, relentless, and it just kept coming.

Get your book written.

What?

Get your book written.

Oh, no, not that again.

But something had changed. This time, I heard it in a different way. I heard, *People are dying. Get past your ego and the fear of judgment. Get past your insecurities and fearing that people won't listen to you. Some won't listen, but if one person does, you will have made a difference.*

It wasn't about a book—it was about a message. Memories of my favorite movie, *It's a Wonderful Life,* kept playing in my mind. People had been telling me for years since I started on the healing path that I should write a book. I guess hearing it from so many people had affected me. I had written down some thoughts several times before but had never gone anywhere with it. After all, I was no writer. Besides that, life was constantly getting in the way. It seemed as though every time I tried to put anything into writing, something else happened to keep me from the work—all of it self-imposed, of course: fear and avoidance, plain and simple.

Get your book written! I kept hearing.

"Go away!" I stuck my fingers in my ears to drown it out. "La la la la la la! I can't hear you."

Then several things happened. It was a pretty lousy time. My father was dying of lung cancer—he was a smoker. The pain of that was so difficult because I knew how much could be done, and yet, *I* couldn't do anything— mostly because he didn't want to do all that *he* could. He made as many changes as he felt he could, but his original diagnosis was very advanced stage 4. The day he got the diagnosis, he made his decision that he was going to die. He was at peace with God and with what he had accomplished in his life, and was ready to go. The doctors told him that with treatments, he would have three to six months. He just asked that I help him leave this world with as much dignity and as little pain as possible. At least I could help with that.

It was still painful to watch, especially toward the end. It was devastating to be at the hospital day in and day out around the clock. It was especially gut-wrenching for me because it hit so close to home—I was reliving so much of what I had been through. I had been there once and had almost died, and if I hadn't been lucky enough to pick up the phone book, I would have died there myself.

One day in particular stood out. It was near the end, and much of the floor was terminal. In the room next to my dad, a young woman in her mid-thirties had been admitted. I was looking at what could have been me. She was roughly the same age as I was when I was first diagnosed with stage 4. She was dying of cancer. It was devastating to see my dad dying of it. But he had made choices and decisions that had brought him to this point, and he was okay with that. I loved him dearly, but his choice to smoke had given him lung cancer. Yes, it's hard to stop, but he never tried.

But what choices could that young woman possibly have *knowingly* made to bring her to that god-awful point? What choices could children have made to be here? What choices could 90 percent of the people with cancer *knowingly* have made to create the disease? I am now aware of how many choices we make *unknowingly*, and unfortunately, most people aren't aware of it.

Coming home deeply affected by the young woman I had seen at the hospital, I found an unexpected e-mail from my accountant, Ed Murphy. I had been talking with him on a regular basis about how he could improve his health and the way he felt. His e-mail read,

> *Joyce:*
>
> *I hope the holidays have been good to you. I thank you so much for all you've done for me this year. I feel great and I owe it all to you. Merry Christmas and happy New Year. You are my guardian angel.*
>
> *PS: I want an autograph on your book. Get to work!!!*

The booming voice got louder. *Get your book written!*

"Okay, okay, I got it."

You asked for it, didn't you? came the voice.

"Ugh! Yeah, but I didn't think it would be *that*!"

So I received the message loud and clear, once again. This time it was about the path I was meant to be on, at least for now. It feels as if I am still only skimming the surface on my spiritual journey, and it is exciting! As I have opened up, I am more and more aware of those messages, those everyday miracles. God had a much bigger plan for me than I did for myself. He knew that if I had something in my teeth to gnaw that might help people—any kind of knowledge—I wouldn't be able to keep it to myself. I would have to share it. I'm not a teacher, but I feel the need to teach, especially a message this huge.

Hope comes from daring to believe in miracles. Daring to believe that you are worthy of one. They happen every day. And I am speaking from personal experience!

Epilogue:

Whatever the Mind Can Conceive and Believe, It Can Achieve

Wow, so after all that, what's next? Where do you go from here? You live life to the fullest, following your dreams, not settling for less, being excited about the endless possibilities and all that life has to offer. You are grateful. You make sure the gift you are given, this gift more precious than any diamond—the gift of your life—does not go to waste. You focus on living and achieving your dreams.

Napoleon Hill said, "Whatever the mind can conceive and believe, it can achieve." I've always lived by that motto. In fact, it might be the single most important reason why I am here today.

Dad taught me that. His unwavering thirst for knowledge was something he had instilled in all his children and grandchildren—that and perseverance. He always told us we could accomplish anything. "I can't do that" was never part of his vocabulary, nor was it allowed to take up space in ours.

One of the greatest gifts Dad gave us was teaching us to ask ourselves, *Why can't I do that?* Then we had to figure it out. For that, I owe him my life. That persevering and questioning attitude enabled me to reject my and Kevin's diagnoses and go against all the odds and against conventional thinking to find a way to reverse it.

The other critical part of it came from my mom. She always told us we could do more. She ran circles around me. When I was sick as a dog, she would say, "You need to read the *Wall Street Journal* today. You have to stay

on top of things so you'll know what's going on when you go back to work."
Of course, I work on balancing both these traits now because they can be
taken to the extreme (trust me, I know) and result in a "work, work, work"
mentality. But now, at least, I'm aware of it.

Once I set my mind to something and am willing to accept the discomfort
of change, pain, or fear, I know I'll be guided. Rather than ask, *Why me?* I
ask, *Why not me?* Why did all this happen? What am I supposed to be doing
with this? No one can really be sure. I only know how grateful I am that it did
happen. This has been the greatest blessing I could ever imagine.

Gratitude is *huge* for us! Kevin and I live every day with gratitude.
Expressing it is like breathing now, when I go to sleep, when I wake up,
when I drive, whenever. At dinner each night, we always go around the
table and ask, "What was your favorite part of the day, and what are you
most grateful for?" I try to start or end every day with my gratitude journal,
where I list everything I'm grateful for, in no particular order: Kevin,
Kelsey and our beautiful little adopted daughter Dasha—see, I knew we
were supposed to have more children; I just didn't know *how*—her giggles
and the way she skips joyfully all over the house, my family and friends,
Kevin's eyes, pillows, weekends, meditation, Kelsey's storytelling and her
kindness, God, how I am always guided, sunshine, cool grass under my
feet, having hair, showers, shoes, tweezers … The list can go on and on for
pages, from the important to the silly. One day we had to laugh—we had
forgotten to be grateful for toenails. I mean really, when you think of it,
they're important. Think how painful it would be if someone stepped on
your toes and you didn't have toenails!

Gratitude is such an important part of our lives that we sometimes forget
what an impact it can have, especially on our children. One of those times
was the night before Kelsey's big Halloween party. We're decorating the
basement, making it spooky with ghosts, lanterns, and spider webs draped
from the ceiling, and an eight-foot spider to boot. We've even changed the
ceiling lights to orange and purple and have a spooky strobe light. It's pretty
cool if I do say so myself, especially since I'm not the creative one in the
family. Kelsey is so excited, she can hardly stand still. Halloween is one of

her favorite holidays because it's the one that everyone celebrates together. She loves when people are brought together. It doesn't have a strong religious emphasis and most everyone celebrates it, so she can say "Happy Halloween" to everyone without worrying about whether it's a holiday they celebrate.

I'm not sure how I am going to pull this one off, since I'm so behind with all I have to do after just returning from a trip. The house is a mess, and I wonder how I let it get this bad. It's clean, just not this messy, but it just happened to be one of those times. It seems as if there isn't a room that doesn't have some kind of mess in it. I have no idea how we're going to get it all done and cleaned up by tomorrow. There's a moment when I wonder what the heck I was thinking when I agreed, the week before Halloween, to have a party for twenty of her twelve- and thirteen-year-old girlfriends. Then, with a smile, I remember some kind of saying about how the kids won't remember what a mess the house was, but they will always remember the fun they had.

I go in to Kelsey's room to give her another good-night kiss. (There are always two or three, sometimes four.) Thinking she's asleep, I bend down to kiss that adorable cheek, and her arms go around my neck in a headlock as she pulls me closer. She whispers, half asleep with her eyes closed, "Lay down with me." Once she's got you in the headlock, there is no getting up. She pulls me closer. So I lie down. Now I know why I agreed to have the party: because of moments like this. She is such an awesome kid.

"Thanks, Mom," she whispers.

"For what?" I ask.

I expect her next words to be "for my party." But she whispers, "For everything—for my life." My heart melts. "I have an amazing life," she says.

I ask, "Are you happy, honey?"

Her eyes shoot open. "Oh, my God, I am *so* happy. I say it every night before I go to sleep. I thank God for everything: for you and Daddy, Dasha, my friends, for the littlest thing from a toothbrush to something as big as my life. I just feel so grateful I have a great life."

Wow. What more can a mom ask for? It just doesn't get any better than that. So I go and shove everything that doesn't have a home at the moment into one room and close the door. What mess? Everything's looking pretty good to me.

I go to bed every night and wake up every day grateful, amazed at all that has opened up for me. I pay attention to all these little things that I wouldn't even have noticed before, like all that I have to be grateful for and the guidance. We live our lives with so much more excitement and fascination, as if we are waiting to see what really cool mysteries await us next—good ones, that is. I am elated when something new and exciting or unusual happens that I know is coming from a much higher place. I get some gift out of every day, and there are days when I am practically bubbling with excitement and awe over our future and this rockin' life and planet. Can you blame me?

It's a gorgeous cold but sunny day, with a sky as blue as I have ever seen. The bright blue sky reminds me of the crisp spring day when it all began, which now seems a lifetime ago. I am terrified, shaking. Am I *nuts*? Why am I doing this? Is it really worth the risk? Can I handle the pain?

Then the reminder pops into my head—what I always say: "On the other side of fear is freedom."

I remind myself that I am doing this because every second of my life is precious, and I am going to live it to the fullest. I'm terrified, but I know what's possible on the other side of this fear.

Kevin turns to look at me. He has that same look on his face that he had that beautiful spring day all those years ago: that *Oh, sh*t!* look of a scared little boy putting on a good front. The same look he wore when he was teetering on that cliff in Jamaica. I can see that he is just as terrified now, and then, in an instant, he's gone. My heart is racing. I say a prayer that he will be okay, that this wasn't just a terrible mistake. His courage in the face of that visible fear gives me strength. I look down in disbelief that I am actually doing this. I look up to the heavens. *Please, God, after all we've been through, let this be okay.*

I push off. The skis feel surprisingly natural as they glide over the snow. Oh, my God, I'm actually doing this. I choose to ignore the pain as I pick up speed and I remember that I have to turn to slow myself down. The cold, crisp air hitting my face feels refreshing, like a splash of cold water on waking. Woken up from that dream … that horrific dream … that other life. This is my new life, my new dream.

The giggles start bubbling up inside me. The emotions hit me like a wave. Tears of joy and gratitude are welling up in my eyes, and I'm laughing at the same time. I am doing this! Can you believe it? I am actually doing this! I AM SKIING!

I close my eyes for a second and imagine I am flying. The wind glides over my skin. This is the closest I can come to flying, like a bird, the ultimate symbol of freedom, of life. I can't even believe that this is my life. As I open my eyes again, I see Kevin at the bottom of the hill, looking up at me—my cheering squad. I think of my own limitations and then look at my husband, who, on that beautiful spring day when it all began, never knew if he would walk again—and now he has just skied down the mountain! I'm beaming.

Thank you, God! Thank you, universe! I am so grateful for all that was put in my path so that I could be here this day and to get to this moment. To be so fully alive! Tears of joy stream down my face, and my smile grows so big that it feels as if I could crack open as I throw a fist in the air and shout, "YES!"

I have spent years making this grueling climb to the top of one huge mountain, and I can't get over how spectacular the view of the future is from here. As I continue on my journey, I can't help but feel blessed for all the miracles I've been given. The greatest gifts are my life and Kevin's life. I am blessed to have this amazing husband, two beautiful girls, and a great family. I get to help people, to show them how they can transform their health and their lives. I have friends, new and old—ones I can explore this fascinating, wide-open universe with, and ones I can just be Joycie with. I am blessed to have the amazing second chance at life that God has gifted me with. I am blessed for all the experiences and the doors he opened that allow me to be on this awesome, wonderful journey to places I never knew existed, and in ways I had never dreamed of.

More than anything, I am immensely grateful for the brain hemorrhage, three strokes, and three rounds of cancer that made me realize how truly blessed I am. Life is beautiful—or, as they say in San Giovanni Rotondo, *La vita è bella*.

Acknowledgments

I would like to thank the following people for helping make this possible: my book, my reason for being, my being alive and helping us reach others:

To Kevin – Thank you for opening up to a whole new, scary world of change and joining me day after day to explore something new and exciting. Your daily encouragement and willingness to support me with all my dreams and visions are the foundation I needed to keep me going. You are a good man and a wonderful husband and father. You have an amazing gift for showering your girls with love, combined with a profound inner strength. I am so grateful for all we have learned together, and that you were given the gift of life to share with us.

To my precious angel, Kelsey – God could not have given me a greater gift than you. It was you who inspired me to keep going day after day. You who are the reason I could make it through every hard day and still laugh. You have always been one of the most special people I have ever met in all my life. Your heart is bigger than any I know, and your ability to connect to everyone you meet is astounding, from the tiniest newborn to the old and wise. Remember all the special gifts you bring to this world. You have a radiant soul; you are a rare gift. I love you more than you will ever know, and I'm looking forward to the amazing things I know you will create in your life.

To my ray of excitement and sunshine, Dasha – You came to us as an unexpected gift. We traveled far and wide in search of you, and we think that instead, you found us. We had no idea the impact you would have on our lives, or the lessons we would learn from you, one of our greatest teachers. Your joy, excitement, love for everyone, and tremendous heart are gifts we could never have expected and are grateful for every day. You are beautiful, inside and out. Thank you for picking us. I love you more than you will ever know.

To our friends and family – We never could have made it through those scary, grueling years without you. You stood by our side, held our hands, called, made food, prayed, visited, flew in whenever we needed you, and gave us a shoulder to cry on. You spent more than your fair share of time in gut-wrenching suspense in hospital waiting rooms and endured the never-ending phone calls of our drama. Our love and appreciation for God's having brought you into our lives to hold us in your generous and unwavering hands has us brimming with tears of gratitude. We are looking forward now to celebrating the happiest and healthiest years of our lives, with you in them. We love you.

To all who have played a part in our healing, have been tremendous supporters and have made possible this book and getting our message out – Richard and Mary, Dr. Thomas Rau, Dr. Robert Young, Brendon Burchard, Jenni Robbins, David Hancock, Jim Howard, Margo Toulouse, Rick Frishman and the rest of the team at Morgan James, my editor Michael Carr, Tom Martin, Tony Robbins, Bernie Siegel, Barbara Walters, T. Harv Eker, Gail Kingsbury, Lisa Sasevich, Kevin Nations, Jill Albani, Jennifer Wilkov, Alex Lubarsky, Julia Lopez-Motherway, Janine Giorgenti, Paula Fellingham and the team at the WIN, Shaney Messner, Jen Ho, Chad Dougatz, Louise Hay, Padre Pio, Berny and September Dohrmann, Irene and Christian, the Marion Institute, the angels at Paracelsus, all the practitioners, teachers, guides, and angels, those whom we haven't even met yet, and to all those who we haven't been able to mention because it would take up a whole book all its own—you know who you are, and we'll never forget you. We thank you for giving us the guidance, support, and means to heal and to reach the people who are meant to hear this message. We thank you from the depths of our heart for your unending support, giving of your talents, time, care, support, inspiration, and love.

And for you, the person who gave of your time to pick up and read this book, we pray that you hear the whispers and find what you are looking for.

ABOUT THE AUTHOR

Joyce O'Brien is an inspirational and motivational speaker and, with her husband, Kevin, cofounder of Feel Great Now!

Within a 5-year period, Kevin was paralyzed after a brain hemorrhage, and both Joyce and Kevin were diagnosed with late-stage cancers.

Faced with their devastating diagnosis, Joyce, an executive vice president on Wall Street, walked away from an 18-year career to begin her healing journey.

After she and Kevin were blessed with reversing stage 3B and stage 4 cancers and other health issues, Joyce's life mission became clear: to motivate, inspire and empower others with tools to improve their health. Investing years in training, research, and study with top doctors and experts in holistic health, she discovered many of the secrets of what makes us sick and how to make ourselves well.

Joyce is trained in biological medicine and advanced microscopy and is host of the upcoming *Feel Great Now* show, inspiring and educating on healthy living—body, mind, and spirit.

A Gift From The Author

Thank you for coming on our journey with us. After they've heard our story, many people ask…"So, what do I do next?"

If you have any health issues or would like to have more energy and improved vibrant health, we want to support you on that journey. Below is what we've included in the complimentary *Choose to Live* - Starter Kit with many of the vital resources we spent years discovering.

Your Starter Kit includes:

- 7 ways to quickly reclaim your energy and vitality and stop feeling lousy.

- Find out, once and for all, if you have food intolerances or mercury issues that may be affecting you and you may not know it. Take this simple quiz that would have saved us years of suffering.

- Our most up-to-date Resource Guide of vibrant health recipes, cutting edge clinics and practitioners, and most importantly, discover the exact products we use to keep feeling healthy and vibrant and where you can buy them.

- Our hottest and latest findings in your inbox that provide you with ongoing guidance, support, education, motivation and a place to stay connected.

Please visit **www.JoyceOBrien.com/StarterKit**
for your complimentary
Choose to Live Starter Kit.

We wish you an abundance of good health, joy and prosperity.

Joyce and Kevin

RESOURCES

For our most up-to-date Resource Guide of vibrant health recipes, cutting edge clinics and practitioners, and most importantly, to discover the exact products we use to keep feeling healthy and vibrant and where you can buy them, please go to...

JoyceOBrien.com/StarterKit

BUY A SHARE OF THE FUTURE IN YOUR COMMUNITY

These certificates make great holiday, graduation and birthday gifts that can be personalized with the recipient's name. The cost of one S.H.A.R.E. or one square foot is $54.17. The personalized certificate is suitable for framing and will state the number of shares purchased and the amount of each share, as well as the recipient's name. The home that you participate in "building" will last for many years and will continue to grow in value.

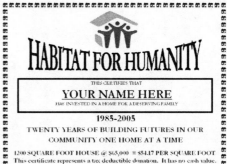

Here is a sample SHARE certificate:

YES, I WOULD LIKE TO HELP!

*I support the work that Habitat for Humanity does and I want to be part of the excitement! As a donor, I will receive periodic updates on your construction activities but, more importantly, I know my gift will help a family in our community realize the dream of homeownership. **I would like to SHARE in your efforts against substandard housing in my community!** (Please print below)*

PLEASE SEND ME _____ SHARES at $54.17 EACH = $ $_____

In Honor Of: _____

Occasion: (Circle One)   HOLIDAY   BIRTHDAY   ANNIVERSARY

      OTHER: _____

Address of Recipient: _____

Gift From: _____ *Donor Address:* _____

Donor Email: _____

I AM ENCLOSING A CHECK FOR $ $_____ PAYABLE TO HABITAT FOR HUMANITY <u>OR</u> PLEASE CHARGE MY VISA OR MASTERCARD *(CIRCLE ONE)*

Card Number _____ Expiration Date: _____

Name as it appears on Credit Card _____ Charge Amount $ _____

Signature _____

Billing Address _____

Telephone # Day _____ Eve _____

PLEASE NOTE: Your contribution is tax-deductible to the fullest extent allowed by law.
Habitat for Humanity • P.O. Box 1443 • Newport News, VA 23601 • 757-596-5553
www.HelpHabitatforHumanity.org

9 781600 378362